Relaxation Revolution

Enhancing Your Personal Health
Through the Science and Genetics
of Mind Body Healing

Herbert Benson, MD
William Proctor, JD

Scribner

New York   London   Toronto   Sydney

o 464593372

Scribner
A Division of Simon & Schuster, Inc.
1230 Avenue of the Americas
New York, NY 10020

First Scribner hardcover edition June 2010

SCRIBNER and design are registered trademarks of The Gale Group, Inc., used under license by Simon & Schuster, Inc., the publisher of this work.

For information about special discounts for bulk purchases, please contact Simon & Schuster Special Sales at 1-866-506-1949 or business@simonandschuster.com.

The Simon & Schuster Speakers Bureau can bring authors to your live event.
For more information or to book an event contact the Simon & Schuster Speakers Bureau at 1-866-248-3049 or visit our website at www.simonspeakers.com.

Designed by Carla Jayne Jones

Manufactured in the United States of America

1   3   5   7   9   10   8   6   4   2

Library of Congress Control Number: 2009050720

ISBN 978-1-4391-4865-5
ISBN 978-1-4391-8240-6 (ebook)

To Marilyn and Pam,
who, together, have rewarded us with nearly 90 years of
married support, inspiration, and wisdom

Acknowledgments

We want to express our gratitude to several individuals for their intellectual acuity, publishing expertise, and hard work, all of whom have made the publication of this book possible:

Vicky Bijur, our literary agent.

Beth Wareham and Whitney Frick, our editors.

Susan Moldow, our publisher.

Stuart Woodward, a consultant who graciously volunteered his time and skill to assist us in the preliminary editing process.

For his commitment to mind body medicine, his encouragement, and his financial support, we thank John W. Henry.

The funding of the Centers for Disease Control and Prevention has been instrumental in making possible the recent research on the relaxation response.

Also, we are grateful to the countless scientific colleagues at the Benson-Henry Institute for Mind Body Medicine at Massachusetts General Hospital, the Mind/Body Medical Institute, the Beth Israel Deaconess Medical Center, the Harvard Medical School, and other scientific and academic institutions that have helped make this book possible. A particularly helpful resource for the description of symptoms and treatments of common health conditions has been the *Harvard Medical School Family Health Guide* (New York: Free Press, 1999, 2005), with Anthony L. Komaroff as editor in chief.

Herbert Benson, MD, Boston, Massachusetts
William Proctor, JD, Vero Beach, Florida

Contents

Preface   xi

Part I
The Science of Mind Body Healing

1. The Making of a Revolution   3
2. The Genetic Breakthrough—Your
   Ultimate Mind Body Connection   20
3. The Fall and Rise of the Healing Mind   31
4. The Mind Body Milestones—
   #1: The Relaxation Response   54
5. The Mind Body Milestones—
   #2: Expectation-Belief   71

Part II
Designing Your Personal Mind Body Treatment Plan

6. Planning Your Personal Mind Body Health Strategy   91
7. A Guide to Specific Mind Body Treatments   109
8. Cancer and the Genetic Horizons
   of Mind Body Treatment   202

Part III
The Possibilities of Mind Body Medicine

9. The Whole Is Greater Than the Sum of Its Parts   211
10. The Future of the Revolution   225

Notes   233
Index   255

Preface

A mind body revolution is under way in the medical world. This revolution is regularly punctuated by research breakthroughs, including our most recent findings that mind body strategies can actually "switch off" or "switch on" gene activity or gene expression associated with disease.

My professional life over the past four decades has been devoted largely to furthering our understanding of the science and the exciting treatment possibilities of these mind body phenomena. For me, it all began back in the early 1970s with my identification of the relaxation response, the term that I coined to describe the physiologic reaction that is the exact opposite of the stress (fight-or-flight) response. The fight-or-flight response is a reaction that prepares the body to act upon fears and physical challenges through the secretion of such stress hormones as adrenaline and noradrenline.

Since that foundational moment, much of my research—along with that of colleagues I have worked with at the Harvard Medical School, its affiliated hospitals, and other research centers—has focused on understanding the relaxation response phenomenon. Among other things, we have established the first effective therapy to counteract the harmful and pervasive effects of stress. We have also explored how the relaxation response relates to other mind body phenomena, such as the placebo effect, a mechanism that may produce healing through belief and expectation.

In fact, we believe that mind body science has now reached a stage where it should be accepted as the *third major treatment and prevention option,* standing as an equal alongside drugs and surgery in the clinical medical pantheon. Hence, it seemed quite appropriate to call this book the *Relaxation Revolution.* But like most true revolutions, this one has taken on a life of its own.

In the beginning, I never anticipated that the physiologic effects we were seeing with the relaxation response—including reduced metabolism, blood pressure, heart rate, and respiratory rate—would be accompanied by molecular changes, such as an increase in exhaled nitric oxide. I had no idea that experts in fMRI technology would find a calming and "opening" of the brain to healing possibilities. I didn't foresee that scientific and treatment links would be established with other mind body phenomena, such as the therapeutic power of expectation and belief. Most recently, I was as surprised as many of my scientist colleagues when we found that the relaxation response can actually alter gene activity—the way that genes express themselves and thus influence the body. Although the genes themselves are not changed through this process, the genetic activity that we have discovered will almost certainly have profound implications for your personal health and our medical practice.

Furthermore, this revolution reaches beyond the treatment of disease to the *prevention* of disease. In particular, mind body medicine has significant implications in the vast, burgeoning field of stress management; according to a growing body of research, stress has a huge impact in causing or exacerbating many diseases. The potential is enormous for preventing such stress-related conditions as insomnia, lower-back pain, hot flashes, premenstrual syndrome, and various types of tension and migraine headaches.

Finally, there is the potential for a revolution in reducing the cost of medical care. Increasingly, medical studies are showing that employing mind body treatments and prevention strategies could save billions of the dollars now being spent on medications and surgeries.

The *Relaxation Revolution* is unique not only in presenting the latest scientific findings, but also in describing how this science can be applied—and, in fact, *is* being applied—to treat patients with specific medical complaints and diseases. Our treatment recommendations, which are based not on speculation or wishful thinking but on scientific fact, focus on a wide variety of conditions, including high blood pressure, many types of chronic pain, various phobias, arthritis symptoms, depression, and anxiety. Yet these conditions are just a sampling of what is possible when the *Relaxation Revolution* is employed in a clinical setting.

Chapter 7—the treatment chapter—is especially long because the list of medical conditions that can be treated by mind body strategies is long and growing longer. This section has been designed for use as a health manual. It functions as a "book within a book," which may be consulted again and again by readers who want to put the *Relaxation Revolution* to work in treating or preventing a wide variety of health conditions.

But a word of caution is in order: In this new role as the third major treatment option, mind body treatments must always be evaluated and used with the same care that is accorded other medical treatment options. Before you try any of the treatments suggested, you should consult your personal physician and seek his or her guidance. This book is not intended to provide independent medical advice or to operate as a substitute for your personal physician.

Also, more often than not, the mind body approaches in these pages should not be used alone but should be employed *in combination* with drugs and surgery prescribed by your physician. With your doctor overseeing your entire personal health plan, including the mind body treatments you may be using, you are much more likely to be given advice that may enable you to reduce or eliminate medications or avoid surgical procedures.

The research cited in this book has been conducted at a wide variety of venues. These include the Harvard Medical School, the Mind/Body Medical Institute, the Benson-Henry Institute for Mind Body Medicine at Massachusetts General Hospital, the Beth Israel Deaconess

Medical Center in Boston, and other leading medical centers around the world.

A further word about the Benson-Henry Institute: At the writing of this book, as the director emeritus, I am confident that the Institute (www.massgeneral.org/bhi), under the superb current leadership of Gregory Fricchione, will continue the advancement of the revolution that began with the discovery of the relaxation response in the early 1970s. The Institute is even now building upon the long history that is presented to you in these pages and, in conjunction with modern medicine, will continue to help you utilize your innate capacity to help and heal yourself as you journey through life.

Here are a few stylistic considerations to keep in mind as you read:

First, we use the term *mind body medicine* without a hyphen or slash. This choice reflects a personal preference that has developed at the Benson-Henry Institute for Mind Body Medicine. Others may prefer *mind-body* or *mind/body,* and we certainly recognize that these spellings are grammatically and stylistically acceptable.

Second, we most often use the terms *gene expression* and *gene activity* to refer with some scientific precision to the new genetic research into mind body exercises. It would not be accurate to refer to the changing of genes themselves, because such mutation does not occur with the elicitation of the relaxation response. Rather, our studies with sophisticated genetic analysis have shown that what *can* be changed is the way that genes interact or express themselves, especially in relation to a variety of medical conditions. Also, we have chosen the more familiar term *genetic* rather than *genomic.*

Third, when we use the first person singular—*I, me,* or *my*—the reference is to Herbert Benson. When we use the first person plural—*we, us,* or *our*—the reference is to the authors of this book, Herbert Benson and William Proctor, or to Herbert Benson and his research colleagues, depending on the context.

Fourth, we have consciously employed redundancy at different points, both to emphasize important concepts and to facilitate the use of the text as a reference manual for those who want to apply mind body treatments to specific medical conditions.

Fifth, we have avoided using actual names in the case studies described in this book and have also changed some identifying details. But we have paid particular attention to accuracy in describing medical symptoms and the results of mind body treatments.

Finally, we want to emphasize that this book is in many ways a current status report on what is possible in the field of mind body medicine. Interdisciplinary research continues, even as we write. We believe that other medical conditions will be added to the steadily expanding array of those that are already responding to mind body healing. Pending work in the genetics field, which links mind body treatments with the healing of specific diseases, is on the horizon. For the sake of your health and that of your loved ones, we urge you to join us in this exploration of the future of medical knowledge and treatment.

Part I

The Science of Mind Body Healing

1.

The Making of a Revolution

We now have scientific proof that the mind can heal the body.

This means that *you* have the innate ability to self-heal diseases, prevent life-threatening conditions, and supplement established drug and surgical procedures with mind body techniques that can improve your physiology, biochemistry, brain functioning, and genetic activity. Furthermore, these benefits have the potential to reduce individual health costs and the broader societal expenses of health care.

How can you take advantage of these revolutionary advances in medical science? The best way to answer this question is for us to introduce you to Caroline, a 47-year-old accountant and mother of three, who started out with some skepticism about mind body medicine. After she became my patient, she soon learned the tremendous personal benefits of this burgeoning field of medical treatment.

How Caroline Conquered Her Back Pain

Caroline, an experienced squash player, considered her forehand her best shot. But as she whipped forward into the ball, she felt something "give" in her lower back. She thought nothing of the discomfort, which subsided as she continued to play. The morning after the match, however, she awoke with lower-back pain that hardly allowed her to stand.

Caroline decided that the pains were somehow related to her habit of bending her back excessively when she was serving. Because she had experienced lower-back pains before—and thought she knew how to deal with them—she immediately reached for an over-the-counter painkiller. Sure enough, after about 20 minutes the pain began to subside. But the discomfort didn't completely disappear, and she went to bed that night struggling to find a position that would allow her to go to sleep.

The next morning, the pain was still present. Furthermore, when she made a seemingly innocuous movement to turn on the hot water in her bathroom, an excruciating back pain immobilized her. The attack began in the same general area, in the small of her back just above her buttocks, but now seemed to spread across her entire lower back.

After suffering the next day at work and finding she couldn't concentrate, Caroline decided to make an emergency appointment with her physician. Her doctor, an internist, immediately prescribed a strong prescription painkiller, a narcotic-like opioid. But within a couple of days of taking the medication, Caroline began to experience side effects, including constipation, nausea, and intermittent stomach pains. Although the doctor switched her prescription to another painkiller that had fewer side effects, the new drug continued to upset her digestive system with occasional cramps.

More important, the second medication didn't help as much with the back pain, which returned in force in a day or so. The fact that Caroline was not improving provided additional stress, triggering the "fight-or-flight response." This physiologic condition, which comes into play when a person is subjected to stress, caused her body to put out excess adrenaline and noradrenaline, secretions that actually increased her sensitivity to pain. The end result was the creation of a vicious mind body cycle of escalating pain, discomfort, and anxiety.

Furthermore, the pain was spreading, moving down into her right leg. According to her physician-internist, this change might be a sign that she was dealing with sciatica. This tentative diagnosis, he explained, meant that the pains might involve her sciatic nerve, which runs from the lower back into the buttocks and the back of the upper leg.

Now at the end of his medical options, the internist sent Caroline to an orthopedic surgeon who specialized in diseases and health conditions related to the spine and back. The surgeon scheduled a magnetic resonance imaging examination, which required Caroline to undergo a nuclear scan of her spine in an enclosed, tubelike structure. The computerized MRI images revealed some herniation (abnormal bulging) of one of her disks and the beginnings of osteoarthritic bone buildup in her lower spine. (Osteoarthritis is a wear-and-tear form of bone and cartilage deterioration that occurs in all of us to one extent or another as we place stress on our bones and joints during the aging process.) But these findings weren't necessarily conclusive about the cause of her pain.

"A lot of people have MRIs that look like yours," the orthopedist explained. "But most aren't experiencing the kind of pains you're having. In fact, most aren't in pain at all. They may have slightly stiff lower backs, but that's about it."

He also noted that he could find no tumor or other systemic problem that might be causing the pain. So, unable to identify the source of Caroline's complaint but well aware of her distress, the orthopedist prescribed an even stronger narcotic painkiller. He also referred her to a physical therapist, who prescribed regular massages and an exercise plan. The new pain medication and the physical therapy helped enough to provide some temporary relief. But side effects from the new drug, including a tendency for Caroline to become drowsy at her desk, forced her to cut down on the dosage. As a result, by the end of the year, Caroline's back pain had returned.

Another MRI and additional diagnostic procedures suggested some deterioration in the condition of the disk in her lower spine.

These findings—along with Caroline's reports that the time she was able to spend at work had steadily decreased—convinced the orthopedist that she was a candidate for back surgery. As a result, she underwent two operations over a two-year period to relieve pressure that the damaged disk might be exerting on nerves around her lower back.

Unfortunately, the surgeries seemed to make matters worse. During her recovery and afterward, Caroline found that she was rarely able to go in to work because of the pain she experienced while driving her car. When she did make it to the office, she couldn't sit for any extended period in the chair at her desk. The only place she could operate in reasonable comfort was on a sofa in her office, but that wasn't a location from which she could project proper authority when advising clients. Finally, Caroline elected to work entirely at home, a decision that effectively placed a cap on her client interactions and on her ability to bring in extra business to her firm—and added markedly to her already high stress levels.

She spent most hours during the day on her bed and found that her normal patterns of enjoyment in life had evaporated. Of course, she was unable to play squash: she had given that up even before the surgeries. But there were other issues. An accomplished cellist, she could no longer sit with the instrument for even a few minutes without being immobilized by pain. Finally, she was unable to interact effectively with her teenage children.

Fortunately, despite all the medical setbacks and the deterioration in her lifestyle, Caroline was not willing to give up on her treatment options. The surgeon had told her that her pains could be idiopathic—that is, they could not be linked to any identifiable cause.

"We've done all that's medically possible for you," he said. "We've operated on your herniated disk, but you still experience pain. That may mean the pain is coming from some other source, some place that we just can't identify, given our current medical knowledge."

That conclusion might have been discouraging to some people, but it was actually *encouraging* to Caroline because she figured, "If he can't find a cause, that doesn't mean there isn't one. Maybe he just doesn't have the knowledge to find out what's wrong and prescribe the right treatment."

So she scheduled another meeting with her family physician, who now referred her to a psychiatrist. Although she was somewhat skeptical about the idea of employing any means other than drugs and surgery to treat her problem, she knew these approaches had not worked, and she was desperate to find some relief. As a result, Caroline was now ready to explore the possibility of an emotional component to her back problem.

The psychiatrist, suspecting that she might be wrestling with significant stress problems, referred her to our Institute. That marked the beginning of my relationship with Caroline and a breakthrough in her pain treatment.

In our first meeting, we reviewed her various tests, procedures, and prior diagnoses. "We always want to eliminate all physical possibilities," I explained, "because if there is a physical cause, drugs or other standard procedures may work. But as you know too well, many diagnostic procedures have turned up no physical cause of your pain. Also, various medications, surgeries, and other medical procedures haven't worked."

I also explained the phenomenon of phantom limb pain. This refers to the well-documented perception by many who have lost arms or legs that somehow the missing limb is still there. They may even experience feelings in the absent limb, including pain. The reason for the pain perceptions is that sometimes, the pains have been there for such a long period before the loss of the limb that the brain has become restructured or "rewired" to communicate the painful sensation, which continues even after the limb is missing. The same process appears to work in other mind body situations, where the brain becomes wired for certain responses, including pain.

Caroline's Third Treatment Option

Then I explained to Caroline that I was going to suggest a *third treatment option*—one that was as well established scientifically as drugs and surgery. It was also an option that carried no side effects and would cost nothing, once she learned how to use it.

"I'm talking about the mind body treatment option," I explained, introducing her to what we have come to call *mind body healing*. "But before we get into the practical techniques, let me make the science behind this quite clear."

At this point, I briefly described the various research studies that have established beyond any doubt that mind body approaches to treatment have a direct effect on beneficial physiologic and molecular changes in the body. I particularly emphasized those studies that dealt with the application of mind body strategies in treating pain.

I also went into some detail describing the nature of the relaxation response as the biological polar opposite of the fight-or-flight response. A major reason for my explaining the scientific foundation for mind body treatments was to engage one of the most important components of this type of therapy—Caroline's belief and expectation that the therapy could have a positive, healing effect.* Because a proper understanding of the power of belief and expectancy is so important in mind body healing, I knew that it was *essential for Caroline to be convinced* that this new concept to which I was introducing her—the use of mind body healing to control her pain—was rooted in scientific fact. Many hundreds of scientific studies have shown that an inner conviction, which the medical community has linked to the phenomenon called "the placebo effect," can help produce healing for scores of diseases and medical complaints. The placebo effect is a mind body mechanism that may bring about healing through a person's expectation and belief that a certain treatment will work.

To be certain that Caroline understood, I summed things up by emphasizing that effective mind body treatments must be grounded in two factors:

---

* See Chapters 2 through 5 for an extensive treatment of the scientific evidence, which I merely summarized for Caroline at this point.

- Techniques designed to elicit the relaxation response, and
- a comprehensive set of inner beliefs and positive expectations.

"For you to experience relief from your back pains," I said, "you must incorporate these two factors into your mind body healing plan."

When it became clear that Caroline was willing to accept what I was saying about the science behind the mind body approach, I introduced her to our two-phase Benson-Henry Protocol[*] for mind body healing: 1) the Phase One relaxation response trigger, and 2) Phase Two visualization or mental imagery. This two-phase protocol has been summarized in the accompanying box.

The Benson-Henry Protocol

PHASE ONE: Relaxation Response Trigger

Step 1: Pick a focus word, phrase, image, or short prayer. Or focus only on your breathing during the exercise.

Step 2: Find a quiet place and sit calmly in a comfortable position.

Step 3: Close your eyes.

Step 4: Progressively relax all your muscles.

Step 5: Breathe slowly and naturally. As you exhale, repeat or picture silently your focus word or phrase, or simply focus on your breathing rhythm.

Step 6: Assume a passive attitude. When other thoughts intrude, simply think, "Oh well," and return to your focus.

Step 7: Continue with this exercise for an average of 12 to 15 minutes.

Step 8: Practice this technique at least once daily.

---

[*] The two-phase Benson-Henry Protocol introduced here shares a common base with the Relaxation Response Resiliency Enhancement Programs that are offered by our Institute.

Option: Use an optional relaxation response exercise described in Chapter 6, page 95. If you take this option, incorporate three essential components:

> *1) A mental focusing device to break the pattern of everyday thoughts.*
> *2) A passive, "oh well" attitude toward distracting thoughts.*
> *3) Sufficient time—an average of 12 to 15 consecutive minutes.*

Important: To ensure beneficial genetic effects (see Chapter 2), Phase One should be practiced daily for at least eight weeks. For the maximal genetic effect as established by our research, the exercise should be practiced for many years.

PHASE TWO: Visualization

Use mental imagery, such as picturing a peaceful scene in which you are free of your medical condition, to engage healing expectation, belief, and memory. This second phase will usually require an average of 8 to 10 minutes.

Total time for Phases One and Two will be 20 to 25 minutes per session.

Caroline Learns the Relaxation Response

I told Caroline that, in my presence during this initial session, she should engage in a "mind-opening" relaxation response exercise for about 12 to 15 minutes. "This exercise will prepare your mind to receive new positive impressions and information that can lead to healing," I said.

I also reminded her about the molecular, metabolic, respiratory, and brain changes that would occur in her body with this phase. With these facts bolstering her conviction that this unfamiliar approach to treatment might actually work, we moved to the heart of the mind body healing procedure.

"It's essential for you to break the train of your everyday thoughts," I told her. "The usual way to do this is to repeat a word, prayer, sound, phrase, or movement that's comforting or pleasant for you. What kind of focus word do you think you'd like to choose? It can be religious or secular."

Caroline thought a moment and replied, "*Peace.* That word should be just right for me."

"Okay," I said. "Now close your eyes and relax your muscles, starting with your toes and feet. Now relax your calves. Next, your thighs. Now your abdomen. Fine. Now shrug your shoulders. Roll your head and neck around.

"Now sit at ease without any movement and focus on your breathing. Breathe slowly. On each out-breath, say silently to yourself the word *peace*. Allow the word to stretch out, to extend itself to the end of your out-breath, so that the *peace* becomes *peacccss*.

"As you continue with your breathing and the repetition of your focus word, you're going to find all sorts of thoughts coming into your head. They're normal. They should be expected. But as you become aware of them, simply say, 'Oh well,' and return to the word *peace*.

"Do this for about fifteen minutes, and at the end of that time, I'll ask you to start thinking regular thoughts. But for now, on each out-breath, *peace*. When other thoughts occur, 'Oh well,' and back to *peace*. Even if you are 'oh welling' very frequently, that's okay."

After about 15 minutes, I instructed Caroline to keep her eyes closed for about a minute and then open them slowly. After she opened her eyes, I asked her to describe her experience. She said she had "oh welled it" frequently, but she had been able to return to her focus word. Also, her breathing had slowed markedly.

I responded, "Yes, and I actually counted your breathing rate. The number of your breaths decreased by three to four breaths per minute toward the end of the exercise."

In addition, she said she experienced a sense of well-being that had been lacking when she had walked into my office. I asked her whether at any time during that relaxation response exercise she was free of pain. Yes, she said, with some surprise, there had indeed been several very brief moments when she had felt no pain.

"Before this, I was in pain all the time," she noted.

I explained to her that, as she practiced the relaxation response regularly, those periods of being free from pain would increase. I then instructed her to do this exercise at home every day during the next week for 12 to 15 minutes, just after she had awakened in the morning, gone to the bathroom, and showered.

"But don't use an alarm to time yourself," I cautioned. "That would be too jarring. Instead, place a clock or watch nearby so that you can glance at it every now and then."

This program, I explained, would help her become comfortable with the procedures of eliciting the relaxation response and would also give her a good start in developing the habit of regularly using the technique.

"Developing the right habits is essential if you hope to benefit from a mind body treatment," I said. "The only way to develop solid habits is to do the procedure daily for a period of three to four weeks. Day by day, and week by week, the routine will help you change the 'wiring' or neurological structure in your brain. Even though the process may seem a little strange at first, you'll soon create new default responses in your mind and body. You will slip into the relaxation response more naturally, as a kind of reflex. So establishing a basic routine this next week will be essential for your improvement."

When it was clear that she understood what was required for success, I told her to return to my office in one week. During her second visit one week later, Caroline reported that the pain was still there, but she said she did have longer periods of relief from it when she was eliciting the relaxation response. Also, once or twice on most days she experienced a glimmer of being free of pain, even when she was not consciously trying to elicit the response.

All this was quite positive and set the stage for Phase Two of the Benson-Henry Protocol: *visualization*.

The Realm of Visualization and Mental Imagery

I explained to Caroline that functional magnetic resonance imaging (fMRI) studies have shown that when individual subjects experienced the relaxation response using the techniques she was using, a calming of the mind had occurred, with less mental "static" or inner "noise."[1]

"In addition, your mind in this state will become more focused and open to learning and accepting new information," I continued. "The end result is that you'll be in a position to make better decisions about your health care and other issues. Also, you'll be able to employ useful mind body techniques, such as visualization."

I rarely mention—much less teach—this second, visualization phase of treatment until the patient has become familiar with the basic elicitation of the relaxation response. In fact, just experiencing the relaxation response by itself is often all that is needed to make significant progress in overcoming a health problem. But some complaints, such as Caroline's chronic back pain, may be particularly stubborn or neurologically "wired." In such a case, Phase Two of our treatment protocol can be quite helpful.

I told Caroline that her mind was now more open and receptive to beneficial change as a result of the relaxation response technique. The technique had triggered healthful biological responses, such as a calming, opening, and focusing of the brain. To take advantage of this receptive, health-enhanced state, I said, "I want you to find a way to visualize yourself without the pain symptoms.

"In effect," I continued, "for eight to ten uninterrupted minutes you should *remember* a state of perfect wellness you experienced and enjoyed in the past. You might see yourself totally involved in playing the piano—a time you felt you were at one with your music. As you observe yourself, see yourself as completely pain free, just as you were before pain became such a terrible partner in your life."

This visualization exercise was designed to help Caroline recapture the power of what I have called "remembered wellness."[2] In effect, this process of remembering prior *wellness* through visualization techniques served to counter remembered *illness,* which had taken over Caroline's mind and life.

Caroline's pain had been with her so long and had exerted such a powerful, negative influence that her nerves, brain synapses, and even her *genetic* responses had been programmed to produce pain. The mind body healing treatment was designed to reverse that process, so that she could become re-hardwired to have more controllable and less severe pain. Using appropriate visualizations following the relaxation response is an effective means to create those new nerve connections and capture the power of remembered wellness.

Caroline began using this two-phase mind body Benson-Henry Protocol for once-a-day sessions that totaled 20 to 25 minutes each. Within about two weeks she began to experience longer periods during the day in which she felt no back pain at all. When she did have the pain, it bothered her less. These short periods of relief slowly increased to the point where she was able to start spending more time with her children and playing the cello for a few minutes each day. Within a couple of months, she went back to working part-time. In less than a year she found that she had to spend no more than about two hours lying down on those days when she sensed the pains might be creeping back. During those rest periods, she employed her mind body healing skills to ward off the pain threat. As for pain medications, she did continue to use them, but in markedly smaller dosages.

To sum up, then, Caroline had taken advantage of our two-phase mind body protocol by going through these steps with her physician:

1. Identification and evaluation of her symptoms by her physician.
2. Evaluation of standard methods of treatment, including drugs and surgery.
3. Determination of scientific support for applying our Benson-Henry Protocol to her condition.
4. Application of our two-phase protocol to her back pain.

These four steps also provide a broad mind body healing model, which serves as a treatment paradigm for the many health complaints described in Chapter 7 of this book. (For a summary of this model, see the box on page 18 at the end of this chapter.)

What Can Be Treated by Mind Body Healing?

Specific scientific studies show that many common diseases and health complaints can be treated directly with the mind body healing techniques described in this book—and the list is constantly expanding.

Here is an overview of the conditions that we address in Chapter 7. Scientific studies have documented that these conditions have improved through the triggering of the relaxation response and the belief and expectation that healing is possible. Throughout, we include scientific references to substantiate the power of the recommended mind body treatment.

- Angina pectoris (chest pains caused by heart disease)
- Anxiety
- Depression
- Hypertension (high blood pressure)
- Infertility
- Insomnia
- Menopausal, perimenopausal, and breast cancer hot flashes
- Nausea
- Pain—general
- Pain—variations
    * Abdominal
    * Back
    * Head
    * Joints and rheumatoid arthritis
    * Knee

- * Neck and shoulder
- * Postoperative
- Parkinson's disease
- Phobias
- Premature aging
- Premature ventricular contractions (extra or skipped heartbeats) and palpitations (heart pounding)
- Premenstrual syndrome (PMS)

In addition to these diseases and symptoms, clinical and research evidence mounts that mind body approaches can be effective in treating many other complaints. These include allergic skin reactions, bronchial asthma, congestive heart failure, constipation, cough, diabetes mellitus, dizziness, drowsiness, duodenal ulcers, fatigue, herpes simplex (cold sores), hostility and anger, immune problems, impotency, obesity, postoperative swelling, post-traumatic stress disorder (PTSD), and tinnitus (ringing in the ears).[3]

In fact, any condition that is caused or exacerbated by stress can be helped by a well-designed mind body approach. Furthermore, because all health conditions have some stress component, it is no overstatement to say that *virtually every single health problem and disease* can be improved with a mind body approach.

Why is it that all diseases have a stress component? First of all, just having a disease is stressful in itself. An important stressor in all diseases is the anxiety, depression, or anger that usually accompanies the disease. In addition, stress may, in whole or in part, be the cause of a particular disease. For example, studies on heart attacks and high blood pressure have shown that these conditions may result directly from stress.

Unfortunately, even as the list of conditions treatable by mind body healing continues to expand, many physicians and scientists persist in ignoring the research evidence that has clearly established the power of mind body medicine. They actually appear to have become *blinded* to the possibilities of such treatments.

Three factors may contribute to this blindness: the lack of profit to be made from mind body approaches, ignorance of the scientific proof, and the tendency to discount mind body techniques as "alternative medicine." But there is another, more basic reason that the mind body approach has been rejected—a reason that is rooted in Western intellectual history and that can be traced back to an error foisted on us by one of the great thinkers of the 17th century.

Bridging the Cartesian Divide

This subheading—"Bridging the Cartesian Divide"—may sound overly philosophical or eggheaded. But, in fact, we in the Western "scientific" medical tradition are locked in the grip of a long-standing philosophical bias that has upset an important balance in the health-care professions.

Modern medical science has long accepted the erroneous assumption—attributed to the "Cartesianism" that arose from the mind body separation of 17th-century French philosopher René Descartes—that the mind *cannot* directly improve bodily health. Instead, physicians and scientists have come to regard the body as an exquisite machine that can be tuned up, repaired, and overhauled with drugs, surgery, or other physical tools.

Their views have been reinforced over the years by the spectacular advances in modern medical science, such as the discovery of penicillin and other "wonder" drugs. But leaders of the medical establishment have often discounted evidence that the mind is also essential for complete treatment and prevention of disease. Researchers, medical journals, and practicing physicians have typically ignored or rejected mind body treatments as "alternative" or "not scientific" or "all in your head."

But now a new era has dawned, as various research teams—including those we have mobilized at Massachusetts General Hospital, the Beth Israel Deaconess Medical Center, and the Harvard Medical School—have used the scientific method to disprove these long-standing misconceptions. For example, our own current research at Harvard, published in July 2008 in the peer-reviewed online journal of the Public Library of Science, *PLoS ONE*,[4] shows conclusively that *the mind can indeed influence the body down to the genetic level.** Your mind can actually change the way that your body functions, for good or ill. This finding effectively does away with Descartes' mind body separation.

Our recent genetics research provides an excellent springboard to launch an exciting exploration of how the science of mind body healing—the third great option for medical treatment—is resuming its rightful, equal place next to prescription drugs and surgery. In our research into the power of mind body healing, it would be difficult to find a more dramatic example that disproves the Cartesian Divide than the discovery that you can consciously "switch on" healthful genetic expression. You may not be able to change your genes per se, but you *can* use your mind to change your genetic activity. And with that altered activity, you can enhance your potential for healing and good health.

Mind and body are no longer strangers that pass in the night. Instead, mind and body have become part of a scientific and medical whole, a complete approach to healing and maximal well-being, which physicians may ignore at the peril of their patients' health. We conclude this introduction with the accompanying summary of our Mind Body Healing Model, which will be applied to the treatment of specific health conditions in Chapter 7.

The Mind Body Healing Model

Step 1: Identify your symptoms and specific medical condition. Your physician helps you interpret specific symptoms and diagnostic results.

Step 2: Evaluate standard medical treatments for your condition. You and your physician explore the usual treatment

---

* Details are included in the following chapter.

options, including drugs and surgery. Learn about possible side effects and also the likelihood of improvement or cure.

Step 3: Evaluate the scientific support for mind body healing. You and your physician evaluate medical research findings into how mind body treatments have or have not worked for your health problem.

Step 4: Apply the two-phase Benson-Henry Protocol. If you and your physician determine that a mind body approach may relieve your health condition, proceed with the two-phase mind body healing treatment (see the box on page 9):

* **Phase One**—*The Relaxation Response Trigger:* Elicit the relaxation response, which will produce proven beneficial changes in genetic activity and stress-related physiologic responses, at least once daily for 12 to15 minutes.

* **Phase Two**—*Visualization:* For 8 to 10 minutes, use the visualization to engage healing belief and expectation and to take advantage of "remembered wellness." Practice the visualization immediately after you elicit the relaxation response—or the time when your mind is most "open" and malleable to new learning.

2.

The Genetic Breakthrough—Your Ultimate Mind Body Connection

Your mind can actually alter your genetic activity—in ways that may significantly improve your health and heal you of a number of diseases.

How is such a thing possible?

We now *know* that your mind can help control your body—all the way down to your genes' activity—because scientific research has proven this to be the case. Furthermore, your mind can influence your body for good or ill, and you can learn how to effect beneficial changes and achieve better health.

Ironically, these genetic findings help bring back into play certain traditional mind body practices—such as meditation, yoga, prayer, repetitive-worship music and rituals, and seemingly simplistic relaxation techniques—that modern mainstream medicine has dismissed or neglected as superstitions or relics of the unscientific past. Many ancient practices and rituals have been rejected by modern science, only to be resurrected from the grave by that same science!

It All Begins with Adam

To illustrate, let us introduce you to Adam, an everyman stand-in for 19 of the 38 individuals who participated in a study* that we reported in 2008 in the scientific journal *PLoS ONE*.[1] The research, with Jeffrey Dusek as first author, was conducted at the Benson-Henry Institute for Mind Body Medicine at Massachusetts General Hospital† and the Beth Israel Deaconess Medical Center, both major teaching hospitals of the Harvard Medical School.

The Cast of Characters

Who exactly is Adam? He is a 36-year-old married white man in overall good health, who was a member of a "control" group of 19 that included married and unmarried men and women ranging in age from the mid-30s to early 40s. The members of Adam's group came from white, Asian, African-American, and Hispanic ethnic backgrounds.

Adam and his colleagues were selected to match as closely as possible the personal characteristics of members of the primary group we were studying—a separate group of 19 expert mind body practitioners. The matching characteristics that we required for individual participants included similarities in age, race, gender, height, weight, and marital status.

When he first walked through our doors, Adam, like the others in his particular group, lacked any experience with, or understanding of, mind body medicine. In effect, his knowledge of mind body healing,

---

* Although this particular study, along with others cited in this book, was designed to conform to strict scientific protocols, we have omitted for purposes of readability the technical descriptions of the specifics of those protocols. Scientists and physicians interested in exploring these protocols and other details of the experiments should refer to the original journal articles, which have been cited in the endnotes. For example, this particular genetic investigation was designed as a "controlled," "cross-sectional," and "prospective" study. In other cases, we have used "double-blind" protocols or other standards. Again, the precise application of these standards can be found in the cited journal articles.

† Formerly the Mind/Body Medical Institute.

the health-giving power of belief and expectation, and such arcane notions as "Cartesian dualism" was nonexistent.

Those in the second group of 19 in our study were considerably more expert in the subtleties of mind body medicine. They averaged 9.4 years of practice with techniques that elicited the relaxation response—such as various types of meditation, yoga, or repetitive prayer. The most experienced in this group had been employing these techniques for 20 years.

We knew from our previous scientific studies that those practicing mind body techniques tended to experience lower blood pressure, calmer brain activity, healthful emissions of nitric oxide in the body's cells, and other physical and emotional benefits. But our objective in this study was even more ambitious than in those of the past. We wanted to determine whether regular practice of the relaxation response might be associated with any changes in a person's "gene expression"—the activity of genes in influencing health or producing other changes in the human body. We wanted to identify which, if any, of the body's 54,000 genes were "turned on" or "turned off" by the relaxation response.

But how might we go about examining such genetic activity? The answer to this question lay in the use of some highly sophisticated gene-analyzing technology that is changing the face of medical science.

Taking a Closer Look at Adam's Genes

Specifically, we employed the latest "microarray analysis" technology to check the activity of *all* of the 54,000 genes in Adam and in the other participants in the experiment. This technology represents a well-established and reliable method of assessing "global gene expression differences."[2] The procedure that we used unfolded this way:

Blood was drawn from all the participants, including Adam, through catheters placed in their arms. Half of these participants were in the 19-member group of highly experienced mind body practitioners, and half were in Adam's 19-member inexperienced group. Next, the blood samples were placed in a centrifuge, a desk-sized device that spun the blood around in tubes until the red and white blood cells were separated from the plasma. As the heavier blood cells of each participant were spun down to the bottom of the tubes, we harvested the red and also the white blood cells, which contained nuclei with genetic material—such as genes, DNA, and RNA. We then froze all the cells at minus 80 degrees F for later analysis.

Each of the white blood cell nuclei in Adam and in the other participants contained 23 pairs of chromosomes, which carried the genetic information of their bodies. These genes and their activity determine who they—and you—are physically and emotionally as an individual, and also the state of the person's health and his or her likelihood of developing various diseases. Every function of you—since you were born and until you die—is dependent upon your genes and their expression.

Later, we defrosted the genetic materials, placed them on gene chips (specially made glass wafers), and then inserted them into a larger desk-sized device, a microarray scanner and analyzer. This scanner, using sophisticated software, was able to isolate *all 54,000* of Adam's genes and also identify which genes were active or "expressed."

Our Discovery: High-Stress Gene Activity

Through this initial study, we found some dramatic differences between the group of experienced mind body practitioners and Adam's inexperienced group. Specifically, 2,209 genes in the experienced practitioners were being expressed differently than the same genes in the inexperienced participants. The probability of this result being due to chance was less than five in 100.

The genes that acted differently have been associated with stress-related medical problems, including unhealthful regulation of immune responses; various forms of inflammation; premature aging, including thinning of the cortex of the brain; and other health conditions that may involve oxidative stress. Oxidative stress—which involves damage to physical tissues by the release of destructive oxygen molecules ("free radicals")—may be involved in various cardiovascular problems, such as heart disease, and may also be implicated in cancers. In such cases, employing mind body healing could in effect serve as a highly effective antioxidant treatment to lower cardiovascular and other risks. Other studies have confirmed that destructive genetic activity from stress-related genes is involved in such conditions as post-traumatic stress disorder.[3]

We continued our investigation by posing these questions:

"What would happen if the participants in Adam's group—those with no experience with the relaxation response—were instructed in appropriate mind body techniques and then applied them in their daily lives for a few weeks? In that short time period, would they show any of the same positive, anti-stress gene-expression changes that the highly experienced mind body practitioners had shown?"

Lessons in Mind Body Healing

To find the answers, we set aside eight weeks to teach Adam and his group how to enter the relaxation response state. The teaching sessions with our experts at the Institute included an introductory session followed by seven once-a-week review sessions.

During the introductory session, we gave Adam and his group an educational overview of the stress response and the relaxation response and instructions on how to elicit the relaxation response. They were also led through a 20-minute guided relaxation response experience, using our Institute's "Olivia" audio disk, a 20-minute CD.* We have employed this disk at the Institute for more than 15 years in our scientific research that has required subjects to elicit the relaxation response.[4] Adam and the others were told to listen to the CD at home for 20 minutes each day for eight weeks.

On the CD, Adam and his cohorts were introduced to various mind body techniques that are known to trigger the anti-stress relaxation response. These included deep, regular (diaphragmatic) breathing; mental "body scans," involving a focus on relaxing different parts of

---

* To order the Olivia CD, which is titled *Bring Relaxation to Your Life*, by Olivia Hoblitzelle, please visit our website, www.massgeneral.org/bhi, and click on the link to the "Online Store."

the body; the use of repetitive focus-phrases, prayers, and mantras; and "mindfulness meditation," which involved a gentle, meditative consideration of any thoughts that drift into the mind. Adam, like most of our other participants, didn't try anything tricky or advanced; he just followed the simple leading of the voice on the disk for 20 minutes per day.

Becoming Immersed in Olivia's Voice

Like the others listening to the CD, Adam immediately felt himself being drawn into a calm, relaxed inner world by the soothing woman's voice on the disk. She first asked him to focus on regular breathing—while letting go of his inner tensions on each out-breath. She also suggested that with his in-breaths he might sense coolness around his nose, while on the out-breaths there would likely be warmth. The idea behind such suggestions was to help him to focus exclusively on the process of breathing and to avoid the interference of outside thoughts and distractions.

The voice then led Adam through a mental "scan" of his body, from feet, to calves, to abdomen, to head and face. He was asked to allow these body parts to "soften" and release any tensions. Next, Adam was told to focus on releasing any remaining tension anywhere in his body as a whole.

Toward the end of the 20-minute session, the voice asked Adam to try counting 10 breaths backward—from 10, to nine, to eight, to seven, and so on. As he counted, he was told to imagine himself on each out-breath letting go of any residual inner anxieties or worries. After this, he was instructed to murmur two soothing sounds, one on each in-breath and one on each out-breath. At this point, he was reminded that whenever his mind began to wander, he should try labeling the distracting thoughts, perhaps just by saying to himself, "Thinking, thinking," or by applying some more specific label to the intruding thoughts. As he did this, he was told, the distracting thoughts would begin to "soften" and finally "dissolve" away.

Expert Reviews

During the weekly training sessions that were scheduled after Adam and the other participants began to practice the techniques daily at home, an expert from our clinic reviewed a home log (see the model form in Fig. 1) that the trainees kept to describe their daily experiences with their mind body exercises. Adam and the others were encouraged to write down descriptions such as these:

"I'm having too many outside thoughts."

"I'm handling distractions much better by giving them labels, such as 'noisy child,' 'barking dog,' and 'uncomfortable clothing.'"

"I felt like I was floating."

"It took me over ten minutes to settle down today."

"I become more relaxed when I'm counting backward than I do when I'm repeating a phrase or sound."

Figure 1
Relaxation Response Training Diary

ID NUMBER:_____

Elicitation of the Relaxation Response		
		DESCRIPTION OF RELAXATION RESPONSE EXPERIENCE
Date:	Day 1:	
Date:	Day 2:	
Date:	Day 3:	
Date:	Day 4:	
Date:	Day 5:	
Date:	Day 6:	
Date:	Day 7:	
COMMENTS:		

As part of these review sessions, the researcher answered the participant's questions, including those posed on the daily home logs. Probably the most common was some variation of this one from Adam: "I keep having these outside thoughts that interfere with my concentration—what can I do to avoid them?" The best answer: "Just say, 'Oh well,' and return to the exercise."

On average, Adam and his 18 colleagues spent 17.5 minutes per day over the eight-week period listening to the Olivia CD and practicing the relaxation response technique. You've probably noticed by now that the technique used by this group to elicit the relaxation response was quite similar to Phase One of the Benson-Henry Protocol that I taught to Caroline, whose problems with back pain were discussed in the previous chapter. With Adam's group, as with Caroline, emphasis was placed on the calming effects of regular, deep breathing; on the benefits of using a repetitive phrase or sound; and on the importance of passively ignoring intrusive thoughts.

But the use of the CD exposed Adam to many more mind body options than did the simpler approach I had taken with Caroline. An important lesson to take away from such differences is this: *There is no single, correct approach for triggering the relaxation response or employing any other mind body technique.* For one person, a repetitive action, such as walking or jogging with a focus on regular footfalls, may be the answer; for another, a repetitive phrase or prayer, said silently or audibly, may provide the gateway to healthful inner physiologic and genetic changes; or for someone like Adam, an appropriate recording, such as the Olivia CD, may be the best approach. But if you use one of these options, it is just as essential to include the three components listed on page 10 of the first chapter: 1) break the pattern of everyday thoughts; 2) assume a passive attitude; and 3) devote at least 12 to 15 minutes to the Phase One relaxation response trigger.

Adam's Acid Test

After Adam and his group had completed their eight weeks of training and practice, they returned to our laboratory for the final test: Their blood was drawn and their gene expressions were measured once again. We in effect ended up with three groups who were evaluated and compared:

1. The most experienced mind body group, with an average of more than nine years of experience with mind body healing.
2. Adam's group *before* any relaxation response training (i.e., a control group lacking any mind body expertise at all).
3. Adam's group *after* eight weeks of relaxation response training (i.e., a group with relatively short-term but still significant mind body practice).

A Chance in 10 Billion

The results and comparisons for the final part of the study were startling and significant. First, we discovered that when we compared specific sets or signatures* of gene expression, or activity, in Adam's group *before* and *after* their relaxation response training, 1,561 genes changed expression from the first test to the second.[5] Again, the probability of this being due to chance was less than five in 100.

Even more striking, when we compared Adam's group *after* their training with the experienced mind body group (9.4 years of practice), we found that 433 gene expression signatures were similar in both groups. The eight weeks of training had caused the gene expression signatures in Adam's group to move close to the gene expression signatures in the group with more than nine years of mind body practice.

The significance of these results came home to us dramatically when we considered how likely (or unlikely) it would be for these changes to have happened by chance in *both* parts of the experiment. We determined that the probability of the same gene signatures being involved accidentally in both groups in both experiments was *less than*

---

* When we use the terms *set* or *signature* when discussing gene expression or activity, we are referring to the specific patterns, groupings, or sequences of RNA and DNA, fundamental genetic materials.

one in 10 billion. It was virtually *impossible* that the similarities in gene activity of the experienced practitioners' group and Adam's group occurred by chance.

Possible Health Implications of Switching Certain Genes On or Off

Further gene analysis revealed something even more important for Adam's group (who now knew how to elicit the relaxation response) and for the group consisting of long-term mind body practitioners: *Gene signatures that were switched on or off in both groups by the relaxation response were associated through past research with clear health benefits.*

As indicated earlier, these benefits included more healthful regulation of the immune system, lower psychosocial stress levels, less destructive oxidative stress, and a reduced tendency toward premature aging. Also, the gene activity we observed is associated with healthful gene activity that is the opposite of that found in many cardiovascular diseases and other conditions.

Finally, after analyzing and comparing the gene expression in Adam's minimally trained group with that in the extensively trained group, which averaged 9.4 years of relaxation response practice, we saw it was likely that mind body practitioners could expect a significant expansion of their mind body healing powers over time. In this particular study, the more experienced group with more than nine years of practice enjoyed an even higher level of healthful, anti-stress gene activity than did Adam's group after their eight weeks of training. Clearly, the mind body training had worked well in enabling Adam's group to increase the stress-lowering power of their genes. But Adam and his colleagues could look forward to significantly more improvement if they continued to practice mind body healing in the future.

This basic genetic breakthrough is by no means the end of our research in this field. Investigations into the genetic nuances of mind body healing continue apace; we are just at the beginning of finding ways that the relaxation response can achieve healthful, anti-stress gene expression. For example, research has recently emerged that enables us to link relaxation response treatments to the genetic characteristics of certain types of cancer (see Chapter 8, page 204).[6] Given our progress, we are highly optimistic about the prospect of using mind body approaches to treat an ever-widening variety of medical conditions.

This groundbreaking 2008 study—which we have presented by highlighting healthful changes in Adam and the expression of his genes—represents a major milestone in the mind body research that we at the Institute and other scientists have pursued over the past 40 years. When I started work in this field in the 1960s, I found myself stepping into a medical arena with the most ancient of roots yet with little acceptance or understanding in the mainstream medical community. Gradually, study after mind body study, carried out with the most careful scientific protocols, produced incontrovertible evidence that the mind can indeed influence—and heal—the body.

The better you understand how these mind body clinical studies have improved hypertension, chronic pain, depression, angina pectoris, and many other health conditions and complaints, the more clearly you will see how these findings can be applied to treat *your* medical problems. But this body of research, along with the revolutionary implications the research findings have uncovered for your own health, is a story itself. That story begins with the fall and subsequent rise of the healing mind.

3.

The Fall and Rise
of the Healing Mind

R achel, an athletic seven-year-old who had become deeply involved in team sports, came down with what seemed to be a severe cold. Soon, she was suffering from a fever of 102 to 103 degrees F and a persistent cough.

Her parents feared that the symptoms meant bacterial pneumonia. Rachel had developed pneumonia once before, and the symptoms had been identical.

The parents also knew the routine. Rachel's pediatrician proceeded with several diagnostic procedures, which included taking a sputum culture from coughed-up material, checking her breathing and lungs with a stethoscope, and ordering a chest X-ray. After diagnosing the bacterial pneumonia, the doctor placed Rachel on an antibiotic regimen. Within several days she showed marked improvement, and by the second week she was back to normal.

Given Rachel's history of pneumonia, it may be that she had an innate genetic propensity to develop this disease. But whatever the underlying cause, the antibiotics had cleared up the infection quickly. Furthermore, her recovery in no way depended on anything that was going on in her mind. If Rachel had lived in the early 20th century rather than in the early 21st century, she would most likely have died from one of these bouts with pneumonia. She and millions of patients have been saved and given a long life because of the discovery of antibiotics—and other "miracles" of modern science.

But these miracles have given rise to a peculiar dichotomy: unparalleled progress in one type of healing, accompanied by a dramatic decline in another. Surgical techniques, diagnostic procedures, and powerful, effective drugs have almost totally supplanted the mind body approach to treatment. Our practicing physicians, medical researchers, medical schools, and medical publications have virtually abandoned the highly effective mind body strategies that center on utilizing belief, expectation, and powerful memories of good health. The rejected approaches of the past include meditation, prayer, the healer-patient relationship, and various rituals and traditions that promoted confidence in recovery.

How did this shift from a strong reliance on mind body healing to a near-exclusive focus on physical or mechanical means of healing occur? The answer to this question is complex, historically and scientifically.

The Roots of Mind Body Medicine

Up until the mid-19th century, folk medicines and the self-healing powers of the human body dominated the medical landscape—along with a powerful and pervasive reliance on prayer and religious faith. Some folk medicines, including herbs and other traditional remedies, actually had medicinal properties that had been discovered through trial and error over the centuries. At the same time, many of these "remedies," such as bloodletting, either did not work or actually caused harm.

Those folk remedies that did work typically gained their power not from innate medicinal properties but from the mind: the belief of the patient and, in many cases, the belief of the healer that they would be effective. That is, patients might get well because they were convinced that the treatment had the power to make them well, and their minds proceeded to influence the healing process.

This phenomenon involved what we know today as the "placebo effect"—the power of the mind to heal through belief and expectation of the patient and the healer, and through the therapeutic nature of their relationship. Many folk remedies in the past worked because the human mind believed they would work. Furthermore, many "alternative medicine" remedies, including various vitamin and herbal concoctions, work *today* with some people for the very same reason: Through belief, the minds of the patients change their physiology, including their gene expression, in such a way that healing occurs.[1]

In addition to the power of belief and expectation, healing resulted from the natural, self-restorative powers of the body, the *vis medicatrix naturae* identified by the ancient Greek physician Hippocrates. Patients in the distant past, just like many today, got well, in whole or in part, because their health complaints were self-limited; they simply had to wait out the natural cycles of their illnesses. Healing, then, occurred both through mind body approaches and through innate healing capacities.

Current research suggests that the *speed* of this natural recovery could be impeded or hastened by the state of the patient's mind. If the patient is under emotional stress, believes that recovery is unlikely, or is otherwise in the grip of negative emotions, healing can be delayed or blocked. In contrast, if the patient enjoys a calm and positive mental state, natural recovery might take place more quickly.

Finally, religious faith and worship, including prayers of healing and exorcism, have often accompanied good health, physical healing, and emotional recovery. These practices continue today among a large segment of the public in the United States and other Western societies. Although many researchers believe that at least a part of these healings may result from mind body factors, much remains unexplained. Unfortunately, modern medical science has fallen short in researching religious and spiritual healing. We may find that the very nature of spiritual phenomena prevents us from doing research with the scientific tools that have worked so well in investigating drugs and various other "hard-science" areas (see Chapter 9).

So these three sources of mind body healing—belief and expectation, the natural course of recovery, and spiritual practices—dominated the medical scene for millennia. But they were only partly successful, as they failed to meet challenges resulting in horrendous mortality rates.

About 350 years ago, progress in developing the techniques of modern medical treatment began to move along a little more quickly— though by today's standards the pace was still glacial. Breakthroughs occurred not by the month or year, but by the century, as the following brief history illustrates.

The Birth of Modern Medical Science

"Jesuit Bark"—the First Specific Drug

A treatise published in the mid-1600s in Belgium associated the bark of the Peruvian cinchona tree with effective treatment for the tropical fever that we know today as malaria. The medicinal substance in the bark was known as "Jesuit bark" or "Jesuit powder" because Jesuit missionaries in Peru used it as an oral medication in pulverized form. The operative substance in the bark was later identified as quinine. Records of those days suggest that the first use of the cinchona bark to treat fever involved a patient who was the Spanish viceroy of Peru in 1630. Word spread among Europeans about the efficacy of the treatment, which has been called "arguably the first effective specific drug."[2] By the early 19th century, French chemists could extract quinine from the cinchona bark, and before long trees were cultivated around the world to provide a steady supply.[3]

Lemons, Limes, and Limeys—the First Clinical Trial

In the mid-1700s, the Scottish naval surgeon James Lind concluded from personal experience aboard British ships that citrus fruits could combat scurvy. A disease that arises from diets lacking vitamin C (ascorbic acid), scurvy produces such symptoms as rough skin; loose teeth; swollen and bleeding gums; physical fatigue; mental aberrations, such as hallucinations; and a vulnerability to various infections. Sailors on long voyages were particularly vulnerable.

Lind, who argued that the British navy lost more seamen "by sickness than by the sword," tested his hypothesis in 1754 by conducting what has been called the world's first clinical trial on a British ship, the HMS *Salisbury*.[4] He divided 12 scurvy patients into groups of two and then gave each group one of these possible remedies each day: a quart of cider; oil of vitriol (ether); vinegar; seawater; oranges and lemons; or a mixture of garlic, radish, Peruvian balsam bark, and myrrh. After six days, the two sailors on oranges and lemons had recovered and were back on duty, while the other 10 remained sick.

Unfortunately, the British medical and military establishments failed to act on Lind's findings, and scurvy continued to ravage British seamen for the next four decades. Not until 1795 did the navy finally begin to make lemon juice available to its seamen, a reform that made significant inroads into eradicating the disease. Some historians have even attributed the British fleet's victories over Napoleon in the first part of the 19th century to the British control of scurvy.[5]

Though progress was being made in effective treatment at this early stage of modern medicine, the rate of advance was hindered by an inability of research scientists to determine the exact cause of the effectiveness of the treatments. Naval doctors could see with their own eyes that lemon juice worked against scurvy, but they lacked the scientific tools to determine exactly why. As a result, there were many hit-or-miss efforts to find ways to replicate or apply a finding, such as the one achieved by Lind.

Because lemon juice was relatively expensive, for instance, the British navy decided to try limes as a defense against scurvy—an effort that gained English sailors the nickname "limey." But limes were not as effective as lemons, and some West Indian lime juice failed to work at all. The result was another outbreak of scurvy among British seamen in the late 19th century. Finally, with the development of more sophisticated research technology, vitamin C was identified in the 1920s as the operative antiscorbutic (antiscurvy) ingredient to treat the disease. The vitamin was then synthesized in the laboratory in 1932.

A Shot in the Arm

Before about 1800, smallpox was one of the most feared diseases in the world. The deadly, contagious viral illness, which was marked by fever and a widespread rash that left pockmarks, killed tens of thousands in Britain, Prussia, France, and other Western countries every year. But today, the *Harvard Medical School Family Health Guide* says simply, "Smallpox has been eradicated."[6]

How could such a medical miracle occur? The answer: millions of shots in the arm.

During the 17th and 18th centuries, Western physicians discovered that by inoculating a healthy person with very small portions of the smallpox virus, they could render that person immune to a full-blown case of the disease. Because medical methodology was inexact in those days, doctors were never quite sure how large a dose of the virus they were injecting into any given patient. As a result, a number of people died. But by the mid-1700s hundreds of thousands, including many in the royal families of Europe, were having inoculations.

In 1796 a country doctor from Britain by the name of Edward Jenner, who had been doing many inoculations with small doses of the smallpox virus, discovered that the less dangerous cowpox virus could be injected into a patient to produce immunity from smallpox. This procedure—which became known as a "vaccination" from the Latin word *vacca*, for "cow"—spread to many other nations during the next two centuries. Finally, a worldwide effort by the World Health Organization in 1967 eradicated the disease, rendering the world population immune. Now, all that is left of smallpox are samples of the virus in research laboratories in Atlanta and Moscow.[7]

Despite these and a few other advances prior to 1850, there were only a handful of valid therapies that we would now recognize as compatible with modern "scientific" medicine. Prescientific medical treatments, including folk remedies that often worked as a result of the power of belief, continued to flourish.

But then, in the mid-19th century, the pace of new drug and surgical treatments accelerated to breakneck speed. With the increased speed came a greater emphasis on new treatments and less focus on mind body approaches. What exactly caused this dramatic acceleration?

The Phenomenon of Scientific Acceleration

In part, the speed of the spread of modern medicine resulted from scientific advances and discoveries, such as the development of sophisticated medical technology. Beginning in the mid-19th century and continuing to the present, Western medicine saw the appearance of the stethoscope, increasingly sophisticated microscopes, and unbelievably complex surgical and microsurgical techniques. Also, scientists discovered countless drugs, which were used successfully to treat previously fatal illnesses. As science in general has progressed, medical science has followed in lockstep.

The speedup also occurred because the general public, encouraged by political and social leaders, started making broad use of the scientific advances. For example, Catherine the Great of Russia had her family and subjects inoculated for smallpox in the latter half of the 18th century, with an estimated two million Russians receiving the shots.[8] Also, Napoleon ordered his entire army to be vaccinated; the king of Spain arranged for vaccinations in the New World in 1803; and smallpox vaccinations became compulsory in Sweden.[9]

Perhaps the most important factor behind the increased rate of medical progress was a set of medical heroes—a group of particularly brilliant scientists and physicians who appeared on the scene to create and run the marvelous machine of modern medicine.

The Miraculous Modern Medical Machine

Three scientists in the mid-19th century—Louis Pasteur, Joseph Lister, and Robert Koch—played decisive roles in launching modern medical science into the treatment stratosphere. Their achievements, which would most likely have been called miracles in an earlier era, eventually came to dominate Western medical care.

But even as we extol the great insights and contributions of Pasteur, Lister, and Koch, who inspired generations of later physicians and medical researchers, there was a downside. Their efforts placed surgery and drugs on such a towering pedestal that other treatment options—especially mind body approaches—were overshadowed or disregarded. Little did these patriarchs and their successors know that their achievements would lead to a near-total disregard of the power of the mind in the healing process.

Louis Pasteur

In the late 1850s, Pasteur, a French chemist, launched the "germ theory" of disease and the sciences that we know today as microbiology and bacteriology. Focusing on the problem of what causes fermentation—including the souring of milk, spoiling of beer, and turning of wine to vinegar—he hypothesized that microorganisms carried by the air were responsible for the deterioration. This idea ran directly counter to the then popular notion of "spontaneous generation" of fermentation, which held that the breakdown of wine and milk just happened without any outside influence.

In researching his idea, Pasteur discovered that heating wine to a temperature of 55 to 57 degrees C (131 to 135 degrees F) destroyed the microorganisms and preserved the drink. Later, he used the same "pasteurization" technique to prevent spoilage of beer and milk.[10] These discoveries had such an impact that it has been said that it was Pasteur who saved the French wine and beer industries. The comment might well have been applied to the wine and beer industries around the world. Also, the purification procedures for foods that Pasteur developed helped in the control of many other diseases, including tuberculosis.[11]

But Pasteur's achievements in the nascent science of bacteriology reached well beyond these accomplishments. He also produced a vaccine for anthrax and tested it successfully in a public demonstration in 1881. In that presentation, he injected a group of sheep and other animals with the vaccine, left another group untreated with a vaccine, and then subjected them all to a deadly injection of anthrax. Within a month, the vaccinated animals were healthy but the untreated animals were either dead or quite ill.[12]

He made similar progress with a rabies vaccine. In 1885, in another example of the type of public show he had learned to use so effectively to publicize his methods, he treated two boys who had been bitten by rabid dogs with a series of injections over a two-week period. The boys both recovered.[13]

Unlike many of his medical predecessors, Pasteur did not have to wait to see his methods accepted. Medical science was reaching a stage where political and business leaders were quick to see the benefits of improving health and protecting the public from disease. One consequence was greater governmental sensitivity to the importance of promoting public health programs, such as measures to prevent the spread of contagious diseases.

As part of this increased acceptance of medical research and discoveries, scientific contemporaries were beginning to learn quickly from one another and even to become competitors in the rush for new breakthroughs in medical treatment. But as they mobilized their resources, they increasingly focused only on the mechanistic or "hard" scientific discoveries, such as the drugs and surgical procedures that could be applied physically to a patient, to the exclusion of any healing functions of the patient's mind.

One of Pasteur's contemporaries—who learned from Pasteur and then went on to make an international reputation in his own right— was the English physician Joseph Lister.

Joseph Lister

Unlike Pasteur, who was a chemist but not a physician, Lister was a 19th-century surgeon by training who also came from an eminent English family with a tradition of scientific discovery. His father, Joseph Jackson Lister, had developed the microscope into a serious research tool by refining the lenses to increase magnification, positioning lenses at proper distances, and eliminating optical distortions. This microscope development and related mechanical refinements helped microbiologists like Pasteur and Robert Koch (see below) observe more precisely what was going on inside the cells of diseased patient tissues.

The younger Lister also had important work of his own—work that in many respects surpassed that of his father. As an assistant surgeon in Edinburgh in 1854, he was troubled by the prevalence of sepsis, a spread of toxic bacteria from a limited point of infection to other tissues in the body. A large proportion of patients with exposed wounds developed gangrene during operations and died. As Lister cast about for a solution to this deadly problem, he began to read Pasteur's scientific publications. The French chemist's work convinced the Englishman that the often fatal sepsis he encountered as a surgeon was related to bacteria or "germs" running rampant in patients' wounds.[14]

Lister hit upon a solution as he mulled over the way that carbolic acid was used to combat typhoid and quell infection among cattle exposed to sewage. He decided to try a similar approach with his surgical patients. In his first trial in 1865, he used a dressing soaked in carbolic acid and linseed oil to treat a compound fracture of the lower leg bone (tibia) in a boy who had been injured in a cart accident. (A compound fracture is one in which the bone has punctured the skin, producing an open wound.) As a result of this treatment, no infection appeared in the leg, and the boy eventually was completely healed. Lister applied the same treatment to another wound in 1866, with another successful, infection-free result.[15]

As a result of these findings, Lister developed a six-step antiseptic procedure to protect open wounds from infection. The routine he established included 1) removing clotted blood from the wound; 2) cleaning the wound with carbolic acid; 3) applying a dressing soaked in carbolic acid to the wound; 4) wrapping tough paper around the wound to hold the carbolic acid and dressing in place; 5) packing absorbent wool around the dressing covering the wound; and 6) pouring fresh carbolic acid on the dressing covering the wound when subsequent dressings were required.[16]

After publishing his findings in *The Lancet,* a medical journal highly regarded to this day, Lister developed methods for applying his antiseptic techniques to various surgical operations and other medical procedures that were vulnerable to the spread of infection. Although his approach to combating the threat of infection underwent many changes in subsequent years, practicing physicians continued to benefit from his insights, such as the principle of avoiding physical contact between an area or item containing harmful bacteria and an open wound. The contaminated area or instrument had to be sterilized before such contact, a procedure that made surgery much safer.

Lister's advances were not primarily dependent on what might be happening in the minds or belief systems of patients. An injured person could be quite skeptical or anxious about the power of antiseptic routines in treatment or surgery, but that same person could still avoid infection and be healed simply through the procedure of killing bacteria in wounds and on surgical instruments and other surfaces used in operations.

Joseph Lister and Louis Pasteur paved the way for another giant of emerging modern medical science during this period—Robert Koch, a German physician who ranks with Pasteur in the budding field of bacteriology.

Robert Koch

Koch, whose work in bacteriology and medical treatment extended into the first decade of the 20th century, built upon the investigations of Lister and others. But he also moved the field forward significantly, pushing back scientific frontiers so that physicians could be positioned to save an even greater number of lives.

While Lister emphasized the use of chemicals, such as carbolic acid, to eliminate bacteria on wounds and operating surfaces, Koch determined that chemicals were actually less effective than heat. In contrast to Lister, who harbored a number of vague or overly general notions about how infections occurred through bacteria, Koch concentrated on identifying specific microorganisms that were responsible for specific diseases. By establishing that a particular bacterium could cause a particular disease, Koch laid the groundwork for better control of diseases.

Another important part of Koch's work was to make extraordinary improvements in medical research methodology. In this role he gathered teams of researchers and organized large laboratories to conduct his research—innovations that brought the fields of bacteriology and microbiology into the modern era. Yet this progress increasingly overshadowed the power of the "old" mind body ways of healing.

Koch's other achievements included:[17]

- Identification of the cholera-causing bacterium. As a result, Western Europe developed a number of measures—including sewage disposal, water treatment, and the quarantine of infected people and ships—to avoid the cholera pandemic that ravaged the rest of Europe and Russia from 1899 to 1926.
- Laboratory experiments about the heat-resistant qualities of the anthrax bacterium, which led to the control of the disease.
- Identification of the bacillus that causes tuberculosis, a major step toward developing a more accurate diagnosis of the disease.
- Development in one of his research institutes of a diphtheria antitoxin, which could be used to immunize children against diphtheria. This deadly disease, which spreads through contact with infected bodily fluids, includes such symptoms as sore throat, rapid heart rate, swollen lymph glands in the neck, and labored breathing. If untreated, diphtheria can cause death through kidney, heart, and nerve damage. Because of Koch and others who

developed immunizations, diphtheria is now quite rare in the United States, though it still may be a problem in underdeveloped countries with hygiene problems.[18]

After this remarkable period of medical innovation, which intensified in the mid-19th century and accelerated throughout the 20th century, many cures and medical treatments were discovered. These included an antitetanus toxin for tetanus; insulin for diabetes; antibiotics, including penicillin and streptomycin; and spectacular surgical procedures such as replacing cataracts, inserting heart pacemakers, attaching prosthetic limbs, and performing intricate cardiovascular, orthopedic, and cancer operations. But some weaknesses began to emerge in this movement—weaknesses that can be illustrated, at least to some degree, in the discovery of penicillin.

The Double-Edged Discovery of Penicillin

British microbiologist Alexander Fleming discovered penicillin in 1928. He observed that bacteria failed to grow on certain areas of petri dishes where bread mold was present. His research showed that the clear areas were the result of a substance secreted by the bread mold, which killed the bacteria. A suspicion soon arose that the substance in the bread mold might be used to treat a variety of bacteria-caused diseases, particularly pneumonia. But it wasn't until 1940 that a team led by Oxford scientist Howard Florey figured out how to produce the drug and use in it treatment.

The first patient to benefit was a 33-year-old from Connecticut, Anne Miller, who was dying of blood poisoning from a bacterial infection after a miscarriage. Such a complication would have been almost always fatal. Although her temperature was swinging between 103 and 106 degrees F, the fever disappeared shortly after she started taking the antibiotic.[19]

As a result of such cures, penicillin and other antibiotics—which removed or greatly reduced deadly threats such as pneumonia and tuberculosis—were hailed as miracle drugs during the 1940s and later.

One of the world's foremost microbiologists, Maxwell Finland, taught me in medical school how dramatic the first use of penicillin was in hospital wards in the 1940s. He said that patients with pneumonia, who would invariably die of the illness, would be cured by an injection or two of penicillin. The penicillin was so rare, expensive, and powerful that the patients' urine would be collected and the penicillin extracted and injected into other patients, and they would be cured as well!

Tuberculosis—the "white death"—was regarded as incurable until antibiotics, such as streptomycin, were developed specifically to treat the disease in the 1950s. Streptomycin, which was discovered by chemists at Merck & Co., Inc., proved to be the first effective anti-TB drug. I can still recall that when I began my medical education, a huge number of the beds in hospitals in the United States were devoted to TB patients. But after the introduction of those antibiotics, the number of cases in the United States dropped by 75 percent, and I eventually found it was a rare event to encounter a TB patient. Unfortunately, an upward trend in TB occurred in the mid-1980s because of the rise of AIDS and the vulnerability of HIV and AIDS patients to TB. Despite this turnaround, most TB cases can be treated successfully with a combination of three to four different antibiotics over a six-month period.[20]

Ironically, the very success of antibiotics, including penicillin, has had several unforeseen and undesired effects. From the viewpoint of modern scientific medicine, a tendency has emerged to misuse or overuse successful drugs. For example, most antibiotics have been used incorrectly to treat diseases caused by viruses, when their use should have been limited to diseases caused by bacteria. Such misuse or overuse has led to the emergence of strains of bacteria that are resistant to the antibiotic.

The basic research methodology that has promoted modern medical progress also has, in a remarkable paradox, undercut the possibility of parallel progress in mind body medicine. One essential line of treatment has in effect made another essential line extremely difficult.

At the heart of this paradox is the role that has emerged for the placebo effect in medical research.

The Placebo Paradox

The essence of the placebo paradox is that modern medical research techniques have been built on a rejection of powerful mind body principles—and especially a rejection of the placebo effect, which measures expectation and belief. To understand how the placebo has been used and abused by the scientific community, let's take a brief look at the peculiar role of the placebo in research.

The Strange Life of the Placebo

The term *placebo* is a misnomer. In fact, the name itself may be at least partly responsible for the distortion of the concept in modern medicine.

The word, which is Latin for "I shall please," can be generally defined as something intended to soothe or calm. Originally, the word came from a passage from the Vulgate Bible translation of a psalm, which was used in the medieval church's Office of the Dead ceremony: "*placebo Domino in regione vivorum*" ("I will please the Lord in the land of the living").

Over time, the term developed a negative connotation as professional mourners, called "placebos," were hired to wail loudly for deceased persons they did not even know. These placebos came to be regarded as symbolizing a useless practice, a meaning that was immortalized in Chaucer's *Canterbury Tales*.

In "The Merchant's Tale," for instance, a character named Placebo is depicted as a deplorable flatterer. At one point, this Placebo establishes himself as the consummate yes-man:

> *And, God knows, though I may unworthy be,*
> *Yet I have stood with those of high degree,*
> *With lords among the highest in estate;*

With none of them I'd ever have debate.
To contradict them I would never try,
For I know that my lord knows more than I.
With what he says I hold firm and concur,
I say the same or something similar.[21]

In the medical realm in recent years, the meaning of *placebo* has become more precise, but the word still retains these historically negative associations.[22] This negativity comes across in two broad categories of current placebo use: 1) placebos as inert or dummy treatments, such as sugar pills, which may be used to "trick" patients into a cure; and 2) placebos as part of established research protocols, which are useless in themselves but necessary to test whether a new medication or other treatment is really working.

As to the first use of the placebo, an out-and-out charlatan—or unethical physician—may give an inert substance to a person with the assurance that "this will make you feel better." Typically, the would-be healer doesn't tell the ailing patient that the remedy being passed on possesses no inherent curative power. But if the recipient really *believes* or *expects* that the substance will help physically or emotionally, the dummy pill or potion may indeed provide relief through the scientifically proven power of belief (see Chapter 5 for more on the scientific evidence).

A qualified physician cannot use a placebo this way for ethical reasons: To tell a patient that a dummy pill is a real medication with the power to heal simply is not allowed under current medical standards. But this power of belief and expectation does explain why some "alternative" medicine substances and procedures have worked over the years—from nutritional supplements, to "snake oil" cures, to various unproven physical procedures and manipulations. Some version of this healing use of the placebo has been going on for millennia and continues into our own era.

The second use of the placebo relates more directly to modern medical research—specifically to the double-blind controlled research model that is often followed. This use has created many misunderstandings about the real, positive potential of the placebo effect for authentic healing.

The Double-Blind Controlled Model

The research protocol for much modern medical research is based on the "double-blind controlled study" model. This methodology requires at least two groups of study participants. One group is assigned to use the drug or medical technique that is the focus of the study; the second group (the "control" group), to use inert or dummy pills or techniques (the "placebo").

But the study is also made "double-blind" by ensuring that *neither* the research participants *nor* the researchers themselves know which group is using the real pills or the placebos. Because both the participants and researchers remain "blind" to the identity of pills or techniques, the likelihood of bias in the study and the possible influence of belief are minimized. Even the hospital or institute staff where the study is conducted must be kept in the dark for the study to be valid. Only statisticians compiling the results can know which participants get the placebo and which receive the real thing.[23]

Up to a point, this methodology has worked well in helping those of us in the field of medical research identify the power of certain drugs and medical techniques. But a serious flaw in the research model must be recognized and corrected if we hope to discover the full scientific picture in any study.

The main problem is this: The double-blind controlled study approach assumes that *any* impact of the mind on the body must be rejected. The drugs or procedures being tested are all that matter to these scientists. They make no allowance for identifying and using any possible effects of the mind on the body.

As researchers with this prevalent mindset proceed with their investigations, they typically dismiss any positive effects of the placebo as having nothing to do with real health improvement or treatment. They discard the placebo effect results as scientifically irrelevant or as existing "all in the mind." Yet many thousands of these studies have revealed that the placebo effect—the beliefs and expectations of patients and study participants—can actually be a significant factor in health improvement. Sometimes the placebo may actually be more powerful than the drug or technique being tested![24]

The Return of the Real Placebo

The scientific response to the placebo studies is now coming full circle. Placebos are still widely used in double-blind controlled research studies to determine whether medications or procedures have any power of their own, apart from a patient's belief. But at the same time, the placebo effect is being studied as an independent factor in healing and medical treatment. Significant investigations have shown, for instance, that the belief and expectation that accompany the placebo effect can provide significant treatment for such health problems as chronic pain, depression, and Parkinson's disease.

So the mind body approach to treating disease—which had dominated the healing arts for so long—faded from view, with the modern medical establishment dealing what seemed a fatal blow by denigrating the placebo and relegating it to a nontreatment, research role. For a while, the healing power of mind body medicine seemed lost forever.

But a few hearty souls—including the "father of modern psychology," William James, and the discoverer of the "fight-or-flight response," Walter Cannon—kept the mind body torch alive in the shadows of highly effective, mechanistic medical treatment. Finally, a wave of scientific mind body research burst forth and began to accelerate and flourish in its own right, beginning in the 1960s. The result was that the fall of mind body medicine ceased, and the rise of mind body treatments began again in earnest.

The Return to Ancient Roots

Despite the juggernaut of modern medical science that arose in the mid-19th century, several prophets of mind body treatment appeared and

managed to maintain a parallel, albeit low-profile, focus on mind body principles. Three who towered above others in the early days of this field were all connected in one way or another with the Harvard Medical School: Oliver Wendell Holmes, William James, and Walter Cannon. They kept the promise of mind body medicine alive, and in many respects we who are doing this work today stand on their shoulders.[25]

The Compassion of Holmes

Oliver Wendell Holmes, whose life spanned most of the 19th century, was a Renaissance man. He was not only a physician who affirmed modern medical science but was also a man of letters, a poet who understood the importance of human emotions and feeling.[26]

In 1843, just four years before he became the Parkman Professor of Anatomy and Physiology at the Harvard Medical School, Holmes published a paper arguing that a particularly virulent form of childhood fever was contagious. He said the malady was likely carried by physicians and other medical attendants, whom he cautioned should wash their hands and change their clothes before they treated patients. He believed that the fever was carried by "germs" on the health-care workers' skin and clothing.

Holmes was attacked by leaders of the medical establishment of his day, who could not accept his theories about spreading disease. They apparently felt they had to reject any implication that doctors might themselves prove to be blameworthy in the disease process. Of course, time proved Holmes correct in his analysis, and he stands out as an early advocate of epidemiology, or the study of how disease spreads in a population.

Just as important, Holmes gave great weight to belief and expectation as a means toward healing. He argued that no matter how *ineffective* a device or medication might seem to a scientist, if a patient believed in the device or medication, he or she could very well benefit. As an adjunct to his convictions about how the mind could affect the body, he became a standard-bearer for fostering good doctor-patient relationships. Some of his colleagues accused him of being

antiscientific in his emphasis on the bedside manner. But he knew—as we have established through later scientific research—that compassionate emotional and physical contact between a physician and a patient can enhance the healing process.

Holmes taught and practiced medicine at a relatively early point in the development of modern scientific medicine. He began to establish his credentials just before Pasteur, Lister, and Koch made their great impact on medical science in the mid-19th century. As the power of modern medical science accelerated in the latter half of the century, those still interested in exploring the healing power of the mind found that if they wanted to be taken seriously, they had to become more scientific in their research methodology. Harvard Medical School graduate William James took over as the premier mind body researcher and standard-bearer in the late 19th and early 20th centuries.

The Mind and Method of James

Because there were no precedents to follow, William James had to make up his mind body research methodology, idea by idea and case by case. From his observations, he concluded that the mind could indeed beneficially influence the body. He summarized the healing power of what was then known as the "mind-cure movement" this way:

> The blind have been made to see, the halt to walk; life-long invalids have had their health restored. . . . The mind-cure principles are beginning so to pervade the air that one catches their spirit at second-hand. One hears of the "Gospel of Relaxation," of the "Don't Worry Movement," of people who repeat to themselves, "Youth, health, vigor!" when dressing in the morning, as their motto for the day. . . .
>
> To the importance of mind-cure, the medical and clerical professions in the United States are beginning, though with much recalcitrancy and protesting, to open their eyes.[27]

One can sense the excitement of James in reporting the potential of the mind to influence human health. Yet, in the last paragraph quoted

above, James suggests the struggle he was going through in trying to convince the medical establishment to take his observations seriously.

James was not one to give up easily. He vigorously pursued cross-disciplinary research in physiology and philosophy at Harvard. Working with two colleagues, he conducted experiments in experimental psychology at a laboratory in the Medical School, which was then across the street from the Massachusetts General Hospital.

James's intellectual and research journeys took him into explorations of the nature of consciousness and a wide variety of other phenomena that today would be rejected out of hand as the domain of quacks and charlatans. In particular, he investigated the claims of clairvoyants, mediums, and promoters of various other forms of spiritualism.

Despite these excesses, James kept mind body research alive, and the profundity of his writings still demands serious attention and study. His work enthralled some contemporaries and influenced the next generation of Harvard-trained physicians, including the great physiologist and scientist of the mind Walter Bradford Cannon.

The Science of Cannon

Cannon is best known for his identification of the "fight-or-flight response"—the hormonal reaction in the body triggered by fear or other stress, with outpourings of adrenaline, noradrenaline, cortisol, and other secretions. But there is more to Cannon than meets the eye.

Cannon continued James's interest in the experimental study of the workings of the mind on the body, including the impact of the emotions. Under James's tutelage, Cannon wrote an undergraduate paper on all that science had uncovered about the emotions. For the remainder of his career as a physiological researcher, Cannon explored how the emotions influence the digestive and autonomic nervous systems. This research laid the groundwork for his discovery of the fight-or-flight response.[28]

Cannon became one of the first modern scientists to examine the effect of stress on the body and on health. Among other things, he found that when cats became emotionally upset, their normal intestinal movements were impeded.[29] In his 1932 work *The Wisdom of the Body*, he revived the ancient Hippocratic term *homeostasis* to describe how the body tended to adjust its hormonal and nervous responses when placed under stressful emotions, such as pain, anger, or fear.[30] Later stress experts, such as Hans Selye, the famous Canadian researcher who wrote many books on stress in the mid-20th century, relied heavily on Cannon's work in their own investigations.[31]

In the tradition of William James, Cannon encouraged his students and fellow scientists to build on his research and that of prior mind body explorers. He delivered a lecture in 1936 in which he urged that more attention be directed to the actual evidence of the influence of emotions on disease, an approach that he felt would provide a scientific counterpoint to scientifically unsubstantiated claims of "faith healers" and "metaphysical Freudians."[32]

Even though I never met Cannon (he died in 1945), I was significantly influenced by his example and landmark research. In an unusual twist of serendipity—or synchronicity—I found myself in my early days of research using the same laboratory at the Harvard Medical School that he had employed decades earlier to discover the fight-or-flight stress response. In those facilities, I identified for the first time the opposite phenomenon to the fight-or-flight response—the relaxation response.[33]

During the past four decades, medical breakthroughs in mind body medicine—breakthroughs that stand on the shoulders of Holmes, James, and Cannon—have arguably become as dramatic as those involving drugs and surgery. They include:

- identification of the relaxation response;
- expanded understanding of the placebo effect;

- linking of mind body treatments to an increasing number of health conditions and treatments; and
- startling "translational" interdisciplinary studies showing that mind body approaches can actually alter genetic expression and bolster health.

Scientific research now shows that the "miracles" of the self-healing powers of the mind and body are no less significant than the "miracles" wrought by many drug and surgery treatments. These well-designed scientific studies make it clear that it is at least as reasonable to believe in the healing power of the mind as it is to believe in the healing power of a given drug or surgical procedure.

But what exactly are these mind body "miracles"—and what is the evidence for them? The following two chapters will describe in detail the leading, scientifically incontrovertible milestones in the mind body field—and will suggest how essential it is to your health and well-being that you acknowledge their validity and make them a part of your personal health-care regimen.

4.

The Mind Body Milestones
#1: The Relaxation Response

As mind body medicine has moved into the medical mainstream during the past 40 years, the momentum of discovery in the field has begun to rival the acceleration of "hard" or "physical" medicine in the mid-19th century. Just as Pasteur, Lister, Koch, and other medical pioneers laid the groundwork for life-preserving antibiotics, highly complex surgery, and other medical "miracles," so the mind body researchers are making their mark with scientific milestones of comparable importance. At the present time, the main mind body research milestones can be grouped into two broad categories:

- the Relaxation Response Milestone, and
- the Expectation-Belief Milestone.

It's essential for you to have a basic understanding of—and belief in—each of these milestones if you are to obtain the greatest benefits from mind body healing.

The Relaxation Response Milestone

Assume that you have one or more of these common medical conditions:

- High blood pressure (hypertension)
- Chronic pain
- Irregular heartbeats
- Premenstrual syndrome (PMS)
- Insomnia
- Anxiety or a tendency to have panic attacks
- Mild depression
- Unexplained infertility
- Migraine or cluster headaches

Most physicians would probably prescribe some medication for your complaint. But assume instead that your physician tells you, "I know a treatment, established by solid medical research, that has a good chance of relieving or eliminating your disorder. Furthermore, the treatment does not require drugs, will carry no side effects, and will cost you nothing, except a little time."

Your first reaction might be disbelief, and that would be understandable, because mainstream medicine tends to focus on expensive treatments involving medications and surgery. But in fact there *is* such a nondrug, nonsurgery treatment—one that encompasses a variety of mind body approaches to healing. Recent research has demonstrated that this mind body treatment phenomenon is so significant that it should be placed on an equal plane with drugs and surgery as a medical option. Like drugs and surgery, the mind body approach may be used alone or in combination with the other, standard therapies, depending on the condition.

A major mind body approach involves the elicitation of the physiologic phenomenon known as the *relaxation response,* which is our first mind body research milestone. The relaxation response has been established by extensive modern medical research conducted and published with strict research standards.

One of the best examples of how the scientific method has demonstrated the power of the relaxation response is evident in our recent genetic investigations, described in some detail in Chapter 2. By any scientific criterion, the findings in support of the healing power of the relaxation response—like those in the following chapter in support of belief, expectation, and the placebo effect—*demand recognition and acceptance equal to that accorded to research that focuses on drugs and surgery.*

The Relaxation Response as Medical Treatment

An understanding of precisely how you can expect to use the relaxation response to enhance your own health must begin with an updated definition of the term.

Briefly stated, the relaxation response is defined as the *response that is the opposite of the "fight-or-flight" or stress response. It is characterized by the following:*[1]

- decreased metabolism, heart rate, blood pressure, and rate of breathing;
- a decrease or "calming" in brain activity;
- an increase in attention and decision-making functions of the brain; and
- changes in gene activity that are the opposite of those associated with stress.

This more complete definition has emerged over decades in multiple types of research. For those who are being introduced to the relaxation response for the first time—and also for those who need a refresher in their understanding—it will be helpful to begin at the beginning.

The Identification of the Phenomenon

My early research at Harvard Medical School with other scientists revealed that mental states could markedly alter physiologic function: The mind could change bodily responses.

Specifically, we found that the use of an Eastern religious meditation technique, Transcendental Meditation, could produce what we called by the mouthful-term a "hypometabolic physiologic state"— the opposite physical response to the stress response. Our research involving 36 subjects showed that the meditation could cause a variety of bodily changes that countered stress, including decreased oxygen consumption of the entire body and decreased respiratory rate. Also, electroencephalograms, which measure brain waves, revealed an increase in slow alpha waves in the brain, a change that suggested an increased state of relaxation.[2]

I coined the term *relaxation response* in an article published in the medical journal *Psychiatry* in 1974.[3] In that publication, my co-authors and I established the fact that physiologic alterations associated with the relaxation response occurred during a variety of religious and secular practices, not just during Transcendental Meditation, which was used by the subjects in our initial study. We noted that some of these other practices included Zen, yoga, repetitive prayer, progressive muscle relaxation, and hypnosis. We also emphasized that the relaxation response, which results from these behaviors, is associated with a set of measurable, predictable, and reproducible physiologic changes.

My later research into the precise biological nature of the relaxation response included findings published in the journal *Science* that showed how the activity of the sympathetic nervous system, which tends to intensify under stress, could be altered with relaxation response techniques.[4] The sympathetic nervous system is the involuntary part of the nervous system that controls such functions as heart rate, blood vessel contractions, breathing, and perspiration.

As our research proceeded over the years, we used newly developed technologies to evaluate the body's physical functions during the relaxation response experience. We explored the molecular changes that this mind body approach was causing, including the body's exhaled nitric oxide (NO). Specifically, our team, composed of George Stefano, Gregory Fricchione, Brian Slingsby, and me, hypothesized that the NO molecule can exert "profound physiological actions" for a relatively long time.[5] These actions include a healthful influence on the body's antibacterial, antiviral, and stress responses. Through both the relaxation response and the placebo effect, this release of NO can protect the body from microbes, cardiovascular disorders such as hypertension, and immune problems. To test this hypothesis, we established in a 2005 study, led by Jeffrey Dusek at our Institute, that healthful NO does indeed increase throughout the body after relaxation response training.[6]

Another of our teams, led by Sara Lazar, used functional magnetic resonance imaging to explore whether the practice of meditation might be associated with changes in the brain's physical structure. The procedure involved placing 20 individuals with extensive meditation experience—and also 15 matched controls with no meditation background—into a computerized, tubelike fMRI device that displayed three-dimensional images of various parts of their brains. The imaging revealed that the participants who were experienced in eliciting the relaxation response through meditation had thicker regions of the brain's cortex in those decision-making regions associated with attention and also sensory, cognitive, and emotional processing. The greater cortical thickness in the older participants' brains suggested to us that meditation might offset age-related cortical thinning.[7]

These studies have laid the groundwork for perhaps the most dramatic findings of all. Our most recent research, which was first published in 2008 and which has been described in Chapter 2, has delved into genetics and the complex new technology used to monitor gene activity. These studies have established clearly that eliciting the relaxation response through any of a wide variety of techniques will actually change the body's gene activity or "expression."[8]

The participants in the genetics study used a number of different meditative, relaxation, and prayer-based techniques. These included repeating a mantra, mindfulness meditation, Transcendental Meditation, Vipassana meditation, breath focus, Kripalu or Kundalini yoga, and repetitive prayer. Despite the variety, *all techniques yielded the same gene expression.* We found that our minds and bodies, all the way down to the genetic level, are built to experience a common relaxation response state, regardless of the technique used to elicit it.

These investigations all highlight this fundamental fact: *Science— the same reductionistic science that is used to evaluate various drugs and medical procedures—has proven that your mind can heal your body.*

But all this research won't help your health one bit unless you accept the findings and apply them. For a taste of how the relaxation response can be used to treat specific illnesses, let's take a closer look at the power of this type of mind body healing.

The Power of Relaxation Response Healing

In a letter to the editor of the *New England Journal of Medicine,* co-authored on October 14, 1993, two colleagues and I noted that relaxation techniques were increasingly being taught at U.S. medical schools—and also used to good effect in treating patients.[9]

Specifically, we contacted 62 medical schools, a number that represented 47 percent of the total number of medical schools at the time. We found that at 36 of them (58 percent), the "therapeutic use of relaxation techniques is being taught in either required or elective courses." We also found that for four conditions—insomnia, depression, anxiety, and headache—relaxation techniques were uniformly and prominently listed as "appropriate," "typical," "effective," and "valuable." In fact, relaxation was commonly recommended as the "treatment of choice." We concluded that "relaxation techniques should serve as a model of how to integrate worthy, unconventional therapies in the practice of mainstream medicine."

Of course now, with the wave of new research, we have moved beyond the idea of regarding relaxation response techniques as "unconventional." The current scientific support requires that they be accepted as mainstream, along with pharmaceuticals and surgery. To convey just how solid this research support is, it is helpful to highlight a few of the most common types of health issues that respond well to the relaxation response. In particular, five common medical problems illustrate the power of this mind body approach:

1. hypertension (high blood pressure);
2. insomnia;
3. irregular heartbeats;
4. premenstrual syndrome (PMS); and
5. infertility.

The Relaxation Response Approach to Hypertension

Our present emphasis on using mind body approaches to treat scores of medical conditions began with early studies I conducted on hypertension. The development of our work with this disease moved from animal studies to human studies to clinical treatment, and it helps demonstrate how the relaxation response and other mind body treatments emerged through a well-recognized sequence of scientific events.

The Hypertension Story

The scientific support for the fact that behavior, including techniques that trigger the relaxation response, can influence hypertension (high blood pressure) has been accumulating at least since the late 1960s. Research that I conducted in 1969 with other scientists at Harvard Medical School described for the first time how behavior can influence hypertension in animals.[10]

In that study, which was published in the *American Journal of Physiology,* we applied stressful stimuli to three squirrel monkeys, which caused their blood pressure to increase significantly. When the stressful stimulation was removed, their blood pressure decreased. This study represented a landmark finding in the field because, at the time, most hypertension was attributed to kidney problems, while behavioral or environmental factors were not at all acknowledged.

Two years later, Mary Gutmann and I co-authored a review affirming these findings and tying in other research that supported the role of environmental factors in the raising and lowering of blood pressure, not only in animals but also in humans. We recognized a link between the excessive production of stress hormones, such as noradrenaline (norepinephrine), and blood pressure levels. We concluded that "[behavioral] conditioning techniques may be useful in training humans to lower their blood pressure in environmental situations. . . ."[11] From here, it was only a short jump to devising mind body approaches that would help patients control their blood pressure.

In one such patient control experiment, a 1971 study published in *Science,* we evaluated how seven patients with hypertension responded to biofeedback conditioning techniques.[12] The patients were connected to blood pressure–monitoring devices, which provided them with feedback involving a light and a tone when their blood pressure was normal. The participants were told that the light and tone were desirable and that they should try to make those signals appear as often as possible. In five patients, significant decreases in systolic blood pressure (the upper reading)* occurred, ranging from 16 to 34 mm Hg. For example, in one patient, the systolic pressure decreased from 213 to 179, and in another, from 162 to 133.

But we still had to determine whether or not these findings could be applied in an ordinary clinical setting, such as a doctor's examining room. The use of biofeedback technology, such as that used in the *Science* investigation, tended to be expensive and cumbersome for the typical doctor's office. That brought us to the next research plateau, where we established in a 1974 study published in *The Lancet* that

---

*Blood pressure measurements are rendered in terms of two numbers, such as 120/70 or 140/90, the numbers being stated in terms of "millimeters of mercury," or "mm Hg." The first or upper number is the "systolic" pressure, and the second or lower number is the "diastolic" pressure. According to current standards, a healthy reading should be below 120/80.

a manageable treatment approach—the elicitation of the relaxation response—could indeed lower blood pressure.[13]

This article was the first of many investigations that I conducted on the therapeutic impact of the relaxation response. My co-authors and I studied 14 hypertensive patients, eight females and six males averaging just over 53 years of age, who were taking antihypertension medications—and who regularly elicited the relaxation response over a 20-week period. In this study the average systolic (upper reading) blood pressure decreased from 145 to 135 mm Hg, and the average diastolic (lower reading) blood pressure dropped from 91 to 87 mm Hg.

Although the subjects in this study used the Transcendental Meditation technique to elicit the relaxation response, we concluded that other techniques would also work. "We believe that results similar to those reported here would be obtained with other techniques which elicit the relaxation response," we wrote. "The basic components of the elicitation of the relaxation response . . . are present in a technique now employed in this laboratory."

We summarized the generic technique we used in our laboratory as including these components: sitting quietly; closing the eyes; relaxing all muscles; breathing rhythmically and repeating a focus word or phrase silently on the out-breath; continuing with this exercise for 20 minutes; and maintaining a passive attitude, ignoring any distracting thoughts. As you can see throughout this book, this approach is consistent with Phase One of our mind body treatment, the Benson-Henry Protocol that we recommend (for descriptions of our two-phase protocol, see Chapter 1, page 9, and Chapter 6, page 92).

Investigations employing this technique have demonstrated the same healthful physiologic changes elicited by Transcendental Meditation. We concluded that a generic version of the technique could be learned easily and would cost nothing.

Over the years, we have conducted other studies involving patients who have used the relaxation response to lower their hypertension. Most recently, Jeffrey Dusek and our team determined in a 2008 study that relaxation response training was effective for lowering "isolated systolic hypertension," a form of high blood pressure that affects an estimated 10 million Americans—especially those aged 65 and older.[14]

The investigation involved 122 patients with these characteristics: at least 55 years of age, systolic blood pressure (upper number) of 140 to 159 mm Hg, diastolic blood pressure (lower number) lower than 90 mm Hg, and taking at least two antihypertensive medications. In a double-blind, randomized trial, 61 patients were given relaxation response training for eight weeks. Another 61 in a control group were placed on a lifestyle modification program, which included education on how to lower blood pressure, including diet adjustments, increase in exercise, and lowering body weight. The objective was to measure any change in systolic blood pressure after eight weeks.

Our results showed that *both* groups were able to lower their blood pressure readings, but the relaxation response patients were much more likely to be successful in eliminating an antihypertensive medication. Or, as we concluded, "significantly more participants in the relaxation response group eliminated an antihypertensive medication while maintaining adequate blood pressure control."

Our senior author in this study, Randall Zusman, director of the hypertension program at the Massachusetts General Hospital, described his reaction to the results during an interview on National Public Radio: "I'd been using medications in these patients, [and] they were hopefully following my recommendations, [but] we still couldn't get their blood pressure under control. And I was somewhat skeptical that meditation could be the key to blood pressure control."

Contrary to his expectations, about two-thirds of the patients experienced dramatic results after they were trained in the relaxation response: "Their blood pressure dropped, and they dropped some of their medication. It was striking. It was statistically significant, but more important it was clinically significant to these people."

The scientific evidence continues to build in support of eliciting the relaxation response as a treatment for hypertension, the most recent evidence being the findings in our genetic research that this mind body technique is associated with anti-stress gene expression. Because stress is a known factor in causing high blood pressure, it is logical to think that changing gene activity to counter stress should carry benefits in treating hypertension. Further research is necessary to establish a definite link between these anti-stress genetic activities and hypertension per se. In the meantime, I feel justified in assuming that this mind body treatment works on the genetic level.

But as suggested at the beginning of this historical excursion, hypertension is only the beginning of the mind body treatment possibilities. Many other health conditions have also emerged as being receptive to this approach, one of which is insomnia. (For a detailed approach to treating hypertension using our two-phase Benson-Henry Protocol, see Chapter 7, page 128.)

Insomnia

Approximately 20 to 40 percent of adults have difficulty sleeping, and one in six considers insomnia a serious problem, making this condition perhaps the most prevalent health complaint after pain. Because drug therapy typically does not work for most patients on a long-term basis and carries many side effects, researchers and physicians have explored various behavioral interventions, including the relaxation response. The strong promise of mind body treatment is bolstered by the fact that insomnia may be related to poorly managed stress and anxiety.

In a Harvard Medical School study published in 1993, our team, led by Gregg Jacobs, explored ways to reduce the time of "sleep onset latency" (SOL), a medical term used to measure the amount of time it takes to move from being fully awake to the first stages of sleep.[15] The usual rule is that an insomniac takes 30 minutes or longer to get to sleep, while the SOL period for noncomplaining sleepers is 20 minutes or less.

Of the 20 subjects who completed the study, 16 were females and four were males, ranging in age from 27 to 48 years, with a mean age of just under 37 years. Their average education was just over 16 years, and the duration of their insomnia ranged from one to 20 years, with an average duration of 9.1 years. The measurement tool we used was one frequently employed in behavioral research—a self-report sleep diary.

Our research method required us to divide the participants into two groups. One group was assigned to a "stimulus control" program only, and the other was assigned to a "multi-factor" behavioral intervention program, which consisted of the stimulus control techniques plus instruction in the relaxation response.

The stimulus control part of the treatment involved first teaching all participants "sleep hygiene" techniques, such as avoiding evening use of alcohol, nicotine, and caffeine; increasing daily exercise but not exercising close to bedtime; establishing a regular "wind-down" routine just before bedtime; and using "white noise," or pleasant background noise, to mask any sleep-disruptive noises that might occur.

In addition, the stimulus control treatment involved curtailing behaviors incompatible with sleep. The participants were instructed to use the bedroom and bed only for sleep and sex and go to bed only when they were sleepy. They were told that if they were unable to fall asleep within 20 to 25 minutes—or if they woke up during the night and couldn't get back to sleep—they were to get up and return to bed only when they felt drowsy. They were also to arise at the same time each morning and avoid napping.

The other group of participants—those assigned to relaxation response training—were instructed to follow the stimulus control treatment guidelines *and* to use a 25-minute cassette tape that incorporated muscle relaxation, breathing techniques, and visual imagery. They were told to practice the relaxation response techniques once during the day in the first week of practice, and thereafter to use the technique during the day and at bedtime. All subjects attended six training and review sessions over a 10-week period and then underwent a post-treatment follow-up one month after the end of the treatment.

Both groups improved significantly in reducing the amount of time they took to get to sleep. The multi-factor group, who had used the relaxation response, experienced a decline in sleep-onset time from an average of more than 77 minutes to 17.5 minutes during the post-test period. Even the group employing only the stimulus control techniques went from nearly 75 minutes to 28 minutes. But only the multi-factor, relaxation response group achieved an average go-to-sleep time (17.5 minutes) that fell within the normal sleep-onset time of 20 minutes.

In a related study conducted in 1996, Jacobs, Richard Friedman, and I employed a multi-factor approach to insomnia that used stimulus control, the relaxation response, and various behavioral techniques. This approach enabled 91 percent of the 102 participants who were using sleep medications to either eliminate or reduce their drug use. All the participants reported improved sleep after the study, with the majority (58 percent) reporting significant improvement.[16]

These studies demonstrate some of the nuances of mind body healing, with relaxation response training being linked effectively to other nondrug techniques, such as behavioral modification, including the sleep hygiene techniques described above. As additional research emerges, we can expect the possibilities and variations of treatment to multiply. (For a detailed approach to treating insomnia using our two-phase Benson-Henry Protocol, see Chapter 7, page 134.)

A Treatment for Irregular Heartbeats

Many people experience irregular or skipped heartbeats (premature ventricular contractions, or PVCs) from time to time. But if skipped heartbeats become too frequent or if the pauses between beats become too long, medical symptoms may result, including an uncomfortable feeling in the chest, dizziness, fainting, or even sudden death. Sometimes a pacemaker is inserted in the chest to stimulate more regular heartbeats with small electric jolts. But in other cases, according to research we published in *The Lancet*, a simple mind body treatment involving the regular elicitation of the relaxation response may be enough to alleviate or correct the problem.[17]

We evaluated 11 patients who had proven, but stable, ischemic heart disease—a significant blocking of the arteries leading into the heart, which restricts the flow of blood and oxygen to the heart muscles. Patients also experienced irregular heartbeats (PVCs), and none were on medications for the condition. We measured the frequency of their PVCs by using a Holter monitor, a device that was strapped to the chest and recorded the subjects' heart activity for two days. As the last stage of the Holter monitoring, we had the subjects undergo an exercise stress test to see how their hearts would respond under conditions of physical stress. Then, we trained them to elicit the relaxation response.

The participants, who averaged a little more than 57 years of age and included nine males and two females, were instructed to evoke the response for 10 to 20 minutes twice daily in their own homes, without medical supervision. After they had undergone four weeks of this treatment, we brought them back for another two 24-hour periods of Holter monitoring and an exercise test. At the end of the study, we found a reduced frequency of PVCs in eight of the 11 patients. The effect of reduced PVCs continued during the day and also through the sleeping hours.

In evaluating possible reasons for our findings, we said that the "regular elicitation of the relaxation response is presumed to decrease sympathetic-nervous-system activity and may be the mechanism by which PVCs were decreased." We also reminded our medical journal readers of the problems of using drugs with this condition: "The long-term, pharmacological therapy of PVCs in ambulatory patients is often ineffective. Further, sudden death from ischemic heart disease, which involves decreased delivery of oxygen to the heart muscle, is common and believed to be related to the frequency of PVCs."

We concluded, "This non-pharmacological method [the elicitation of the relaxation response] associated with decreased PVCs in most patients investigated may therefore prove to be most useful and significant." Given the fact that PVCs are sometimes triggered by high-pressure, stressful situations—and that stressful genetic expression can be changed with the relaxation response—we would recommend that you consider a similar mind body approach if you experience irregular heartbeats. (For a detailed approach to treating irregular heartbeats and palpitations, or pounding heartbeats, using our two-phase Benson-Henry Protocol, see Chapter 7, page 190.)

Solving the PMS Puzzle

Premenstrual syndrome (PMS) is a condition that can occur between a woman's ovulation and menstruation when the ovaries are making progesterone. PMS afflicts at least 75 percent of women who ovulate, and may be accompanied by a variety of uncomfortable symptoms. On the physical level, these may include fatigue, cravings for sweet or salty foods, abdominal bloating and pain, swollen hands or feet, tender breasts, and gastrointestinal upsets. Emotionally, women with PMS may experience depression, irritability, mood swings, and impairment of concentration and memory.[18]

Nancy Rigotti, of the Massachusetts General Hospital and the Harvard Medical School, wrote in the *Harvard Medical School Family Health Guide* that women with PMS should include as part of their treatment a focus on improving "lifestyle factors." These factors include getting regular aerobic exercise; avoiding caffeine, alcohol, salt, and sweets; and "practicing stress-reduction techniques such as the relaxation response."[19] She made these recommendations several years before our genetic research, published in 2008, clarified more precisely the mechanism of the relaxation response.

A scientific source for Rigotti's recommendation can be found in an article authored by Irene Goodale and our team in 1990 in *Obstetrics & Gynecology*. The research involved a five-month study of 46 women who were suffering from PMS.[20] We divided the women into three groups. One group only kept daily charts of their symptoms; the second group did leisure reading for a few minutes twice a day, in addition to charting their own symptoms; and the third group learned to elicit the relaxation response twice a day, in addition to charting symptoms.

At the end of the study, the relaxation response group showed significantly greater improvement than the other two groups. In women with the most severe symptoms, the relaxation response showed a 58 percent improvement, as compared with a 27 percent improvement for the casual reading group and a 17 percent improvement for the group that only charted their symptoms.

We concluded that "regular elicitation of the relaxation response is an effective treatment for physical and emotional premenstrual symptoms, and is most effective in women with severe symptoms."

(For a detailed approach to treating PMS using our two-phase Benson-Henry Protocol, see Chapter 7, page 197.)

Infertility

A number of drugs and surgical procedures may be effective treatments for infertility. But do not overlook ways to improve fertility "naturally," says Alice Domar of Beth Israel Deaconess Medical Center and the Harvard Medical School. In the *Harvard Medical School Family Health Guide,* she lists a number of these natural methods, such as avoiding alcohol and giving up smoking, and ends with this recommendation for patients: "Reduce stress"—referring readers to a section of the *Guide* where I describe the basic technique to elicit the relaxation response.[21]

Support for Domar's advice can be found in research she conducted in 1990 with Machelle M. Seibel and me at Harvard Medical School, the New England Deaconess Hospital, and Beth Israel Hospital. In that study, we enrolled 54 women—all infertile for an average of 3.3 years—in a 10-week program where they learned to elicit the relaxation response and manage their life stress in a variety of other ways.

Within six months of completing the program, 34 percent of the women became pregnant, a result that we concluded "established a role for stress reduction in the long-term treatment of infertility." We recommended that this behavioral treatment be considered for infertile couples "before or in conjunction with reproductive technologies

such as intrauterine insemination and gamete intrafallopian trans-
fer."[22]

(For a detailed approach to treating infertility using our two-phase
Benson-Henry Protocol, see Chapter 7, page 132.)

These are just a few medical highlights that illustrate what is possible
with relaxation response healing. The findings represent only a taste
of the full potential of mind body medicine. To understand further
how this process works, we must now explore in greater depth the
second major milestone in effective mind body healing: the power of
expectation-belief.

5.

The Mind Body Milestones
#2: Expectation-Belief

T he power of expectation—the kind of expectation that embraces a deep belief that what is expected will actually occur—has long been recognized as a significant mental and emotional force. Shakespeare wrote:

> I am giddy, expectation whirls me round.
> The imaginary relish is so sweet
> That it enchants my sense.[1]

Likewise, belief itself—or at least belief in those things that are regarded as good and true—has consistently been extolled as a great virtue. The 17th-century English philosopher and essayist Sir Francis Bacon declared that "the belief of truth, which is the enjoying of it, is the sovereign good of human nature."[2]

But is there any scientific foundation for placing expectation and belief on such a high pedestal? More specifically and personally, just how powerful can your personal beliefs and expectations be in the healing process?

Let's allow a 2002 study in the *New England Journal of Medicine*[3] to suggest an answer.

How Powerful Are Expectation and Belief?

In this study, conducted by scientists at the Baylor College of Medicine, 165 patients with osteoarthritis (wear-and-tear arthritis) of the knee randomly received one of three treatments:

- arthroscopic debridement (removal of dead tissue inside the knee);
- arthroscopic lavage (washing-out of the knee joint); or
- placebo "sham" surgery.

Arthroscopy involves the use of a fiber-optic device that is inserted to permit observation of the inside of a joint and to facilitate surgical procedures inside the joint. In this investigation, the placebo surgery involved having a physician make a surface skin incision on the knee and simulate a debridement without insertion of an arthroscope.*

The researchers assessed the outcomes of the procedures over a 24-month period. The results were startling: The investigators reported that at no point did the patients who had the real surgery have less knee pain or better physical function than the placebo group. *The sham surgery worked as well as the real surgery.*

The researchers concluded that there was no clinically meaningful difference among the three groups. In fact, they said, at some points during follow-up, objective physical function of the patients was significantly *worse* in the debridement group than in the placebo group!

---

* For a fuller description of this study, including the consent procedures for patients, see Chapter 7, page 165. The methodology of using sham surgery continues to be controversial, as we have noted elsewhere. The rationale is that it is acceptable to use this approach so long as patients are fully informed that they may or may not receive surgery and also that they will have the opportunity to receive the real treatment (provided it has proven effective) after the experiment is finished.

This study is by no means an isolated example of the power of belief and expectation. Hundreds of other investigations, involving a wide variety of diseases and health problems, have demonstrated the power of the human mind over disease. The treatment principle might be summed up this way:

> Just as an antibiotic drug may stop an infection or surgery may eliminate a malignancy, so the mind—your mind—has the capacity to treat or even cure many of your serious physical and emotional complaints.

Let's make this even more personal. Ask yourself: "Do I really *believe* this principle?"

If you can answer, "Yes, I believe it," then you are at least halfway to your final destination: the healing frame of mind that enables you to learn, accept, and apply established mind body treatments for dozens of diseases and health conditions. The chances are, however, that you still have some doubts.

The End of Doubt

Why is it so hard sometimes to accept the clear facts about mind body healing? Two common reasons come to mind: 1) You may lack support from a personal physician or other medical adviser, who may be ignorant of mind body approaches to treatment. 2) You may be trapped in an overly narrow mindset that makes it difficult or impossible for you to believe the scientific evidence that mind body healing will really work.

The Personal Physician Issue

You may be skeptical about mind body techniques because your personal health-care professional lacks an understanding of mind body research. Your family physician or medical specialist may do a great job monitoring the condition of your heart, colon, kidneys, uterus, or prostate and prescribing appropriate medications and lifestyle changes to reduce your risk levels. But he or she may have serious reservations about mind body medicine, despite the evidence.

This book has been designed to help you collaborate with your personal physician in finding and applying effective mind body approaches to various illnesses. Because mind body treatments are unfamiliar to many practicing physicians, you may have to spend some time in dialogue with your doctor about pursuing this treatment approach.

The Narrow—Reductionistic—Mindset

To banish your doubts and gain access to mind body healing, you may have to change some of your basic assumptions about medical treatment. Reductionism simply refers to the tendency to try to explain or reduce complex life processes to simplistic, mechanical, or very limited components. Medical reductionism involves a basic assumption that only certain specific physical treatments will be effective in responding to illnesses and conditions.

For example, like most patients and physicians these days, you may be trapped in a restricted, reductionistic mindset that says, "A *real* cure for a serious illness is possible only through drugs, surgery, or some other physical procedure. Any suggested treatment apart from these physical responses is 'unscientific' and will probably be ineffective."

To escape this limited view of healing—and doubts about the potential of mind body medicine—join us now in examining the evidence for belief as an essential factor in your approach to the treatment of disease.

The Meaning of Belief

The first step in appropriating the great power of belief in your personal health-care plan is to understand what we mean when we use the term *belief*. A helpful approach for many people is to distinguish between two major types of belief: 1) scientific expectation-belief, and 2) spiritual belief. Although the two may at times overlap, the distinction is important to keep in mind when medical treatment is involved.

Scientific Expectation-Belief

This first type of belief involves an acceptance of scientific research that establishes the power of the mind to influence the body. Despite the vast body of published findings, many physicians and patients simply cannot bring themselves to believe their eyes and ears when mind body research is reported. Perhaps you have read or heard news accounts of how the mind can heal the body, but you have found that you lack confidence in applying these research findings to improve your health. Or a nagging doubt says, "This can't be real scientific research—because it deals with things that are happening in the head, not the body."

In the following pages you will learn how to correct such misconceptions—and use the medical proofs of mind body healing to eliminate your doubts and incorporate the healing power of belief in the validity of this type of scientific research.

Spiritual Belief

A second type of belief—which encompasses various religious or other traditions that affirm faith in a "higher power"—lies mostly beyond the scope of this book. By definition, spiritual belief exists largely outside our reductionistic scientific tools and understanding.

Certainly, research is proceeding on several fronts to explore how the scientific method can measure, at least in part, the healing that occurs through the exercise of religious disciplines and worship or related practices. But so far, we have little indication that science can go very far in unveiling the mysteries of spirituality.

On the other hand, a religious faith or other deep personal

conviction can play an important role in reinforcing what we are calling "scientific" expectation-belief. Throughout the treatment section of this book (Part II), for instance, we encourage those with a spiritual orientation to bring their worldview into play as they apply mind body techniques to their medical problems and complaints. Specifically, we have discovered that in eliciting the relaxation response (what we call "Phase One" of the Benson-Henry Protocol— see Chapter 1, page 9, and Chapter 6, page 92), the choice of a focus word that is associated with your personal belief system can bolster the healing potential of the focus word or prayer. Also, relying on your belief system in employing the visualization part of your mind body treatment ("Phase Two" of our mind body treatment protocol—again, see Chapters 1 and 6) can enhance the efficacy of that visualization.

But what is the nature of this expectation-belief that plays such an important role in mind body medicine? To answer, we now turn to a more detailed discussion of the scientific foundations of the Expectation-Belief Milestone.

The Expectation-Belief Milestone

Scientific research involving the Expectation-Belief Milestone has been conducted on a wide variety of diseases that have been helped or cured by a deep conviction or firm expectation that a particular treatment will produce healing. Over the centuries, a key player in this expectation-belief scenario has been the placebo effect, which has been employed effectively by folk healers, as well as physicians who, in the past—before ethical sensitivities were sharpened—prescribed sugar pills and dummy treatments not designed to have an impact physically or chemically. As we have already seen, contemporary medical researchers have used the placebo to design controlled research trials. But scientific research over the past four decades has made it clear that there is much more to the expectation-belief mechanism than what many practicing physicians and medical researchers have assumed.

The Broad Nature of Expectation-Belief

To indicate the broad scope of this particular milestone, we have labeled this category "expectation-belief"—but even that term doesn't do justice to this powerful, wide-ranging healing mechanism.[4] The mind body research in this area may encompass one or more of these belief-related phenomena:

- a belief of the patient that a particular treatment can work;
- a belief of the healer/physician that a particular treatment can work;
- a trusting relationship between the patient and the healer—a belief in each other;
- a sense of expectancy—or a highly positive, future-oriented mindset—that a particular approach to healing will improve or cure a particular disease or symptom.

As these expectation-belief factors come into play in the mind and emotions, healthful physiologic changes occur in the body, all the way down to the molecular level. For example, the scientific evidence shows that the body's output of nitric oxide—a molecule associated with good health, including antibacterial and antiviral responses and also beneficial changes in the cardiovascular system—can be induced by the placebo effect.[5]

But while the nitric oxide emissions remain hidden from all except scientists with sophisticated measuring instruments, the healing power of the internal expectation-belief mechanism may become quite evident to the researcher—and also to the physician and patient in the examining room. A few illustrations from recent scientific investigations show how belief and expectation have relieved a number of serious symptoms.

Belief Over Pain

One of the most consistent and dramatic impacts of expectation-belief in improving health is to counter pain, including chronic pain.

Italian scientists, publishing their research in 2003 in the *Journal of Neuroscience,*[6] studied 60 healthy volunteers who signed a consent form agreeing to have a brief tourniquet procedure on the arm. While experiencing pain from the tourniquet, each group of the volunteers received a different treatment from the researchers over the four days of the study:

- One group received no treatment.
- A second group received an injection of an inert saline (salt) solution, which the group was told was a powerful painkiller.
- A third group received a saline injection, which the researchers said was a drug that increased pain.
- A fourth group was treated with a painkiller, ketorolac tromethamine, on the second and third day of the study but then received an inert injection of saline on the fourth day—with the verbal suggestion that this injection was a real painkiller.
- A fifth group was treated with the painkiller ketorolac on the second and third days and then received an injection of inert saline on the fourth day, but this time with the verbal suggestion that it was a drug that increased pain.

The results of this study confirmed what we know about the healing power of belief, expectation, and the placebo effect. When participants were given the inert saline solution and were told that it would *reduce* pain, a significant reduction in their perceived pain did indeed occur. Conversely, those participants who were told that the saline solution would *increase* their pain actually did experience an increase in pain.

When participants received the painkiller ketorolac *plus* a suggestion that the inert saline solution would reduce the pain, their pain tolerance was considerably greater than the pain tolerance of those who got the inert saline solution (the placebo) alone. So the best treatment in this case was a *combination treatment* of the real painkiller *and* the expectation of relief. We have seen this interesting result in the use of other drugs as well.

The researchers concluded that "verbally induced expectation plays a crucial role in each of these experimental conditions, even after the pharmacological preconditioning with ketorolac."

In a related review article in the *Journal of Neuroscience* in 2005, the lead researcher in the above Italian study, Fabrizio Benedetti, collaborated with scientists from Emory University, Columbia University, the University of Maryland, and the University of Michigan. These experts confirmed that the placebo effect—with an emphasis on belief and expectation of pain relief—operates in the body through the release of natural opioid mechanisms, which alleviate pain. These mechanisms include an increase in the concentration of neurotransmitters (endorphins)* in chronic pain patients who were able to avail themselves of the power of belief and expectation in pain relief.[7] The body's release of endorphins has long been associated with feelings of well-being and reduced pain, and may accompany such activities as aerobic exercise.

An Answer to Angina Pectoris

A study I conducted at Boston's Beth Israel Hospital with David P. McCallie, Jr., published in 1979 in the *New England Journal of Medicine,*

---

* Neurotransmitters are chemical agents that send nerve impulses across synapses, or linkages between neurons (nerve cells). Properly functioning neurotransmitters are associated with a healthy nervous system.

focused on how the placebo effect could reduce angina pectoris (chest pains associated with diminished flow of blood to the heart muscles).[8] These early findings have held up well in clinical applications in subsequent years: I still find, 30 years later, that the two-phase Benson-Henry Protocol described in this book works well in helping many patients with angina pains.

In our investigation, we analyzed data from 13 studies involving 1,187 patients who had used five different inactive treatments over a period of four decades. The five treatments for angina pectoris that we examined were believed at various times to be effective treatments for this type of chest pain but were later shown to have no underlying physiologic basis of healing. These ineffectual treatments included various types of drug therapies, which were later proven to have no pain-relieving properties. Also, we looked at different useless surgical procedures that had been performed in an attempt to relieve the pain, including the ligation, or tying off, of one of the small arteries of the chest, the internal mammary artery.

An interesting aspect of our findings was that the inert substances or surgeries—which patients and *also physician-researchers* truly believed would alleviate pain—typically reduced pain in 70 to 90 percent of patients when they were first applied. But when other physician-researchers began to question or disbelieve the efficacy of the treatments, the effectiveness rate decreased to 30 to 40 percent. Belief by the researcher applying the treatments led to significant relief from chest pains; skepticism in the researcher, however, greatly reduced the patient's relief from the pain. Clearly, the belief of the physician in the cure can make a huge difference in treatment outcome!

The problem with many of the early studies we evaluated in this report was that their method of application would be prohibited today as unethical, primarily because the patients in the studies did not participate with informed consent. Certainly, a physician in a private examining room cannot simply give a dummy pill to a patient and say, "This is a good treatment for your chest pain." Similarly, a surgeon in an ordinary operating setting cannot try a genuine procedure in one patient and employ nothing more than a skin incision in another to test whether or not the genuine procedure really works. Yet both these methods were used to good effect by the early researchers we evaluated. If they can be replicated ethically, they become powerful treatment tools. Such replication has been our objective in the practical treatment recommendations in Chapter 7.

So the question remains: How can the impressive expectation-belief power of the placebo effect—which we identified in an average of 82.4 percent of the early-stage patients in our angina investigation—be captured as a painkilling treatment option without tricking or harming the average patient with an invasive procedure? The answer to this question comprises a large part of Chapter 7, which contains practical strategies of mind body healing. (For a detailed approach to treating angina pectoris using our two-phase Benson-Henry Protocol, see Chapter 7, page 112.)

Dealing with Depression

Another major health concern, depression, also has responded well to the power of the placebo effect. Currently, more than 20 million Americans suffer from depression, according to the National Institutes of Health.[9] But a number of researchers have recognized that depression could be alleviated in up to 50 percent of patients not just by the common remedy, drugs, but by the expectation and belief associated with the placebo effect.[10]

A mechanism that contributes to this power of the placebo in depression involves the release of the neurotransmitter serotonin, which must be present in sufficient quantities in the body to ward off depressive states.[11] Researchers have determined through sophisticated brain research technology that when the placebo effect results in recovery from depression, specific changes occur in the brain in frontal and cingulate cortical activity.[12] These parts of the brain have been associated with the presence or absence of depression.

Researchers into depression actually seem to become befuddled, because often they discover that much of the positive response of patients to antidepressant medication is the result of the expectation-belief features of the placebo response.[13]

Furthermore, the impact of the placebo on depression is not a short-lived phenomenon. A 2008 review article in the *Journal of Psychiatric Research* showed that, in eight placebo-controlled antidepressant trials involving 3,063 depressed patients, 79 percent receiving the placebo experienced a lessening of their depressive symptoms and suffered no relapse while undergoing more than 12 weeks of placebo treatment.[14]

The treatment that the placebo-taking patients received had no pharmaceutical component and involved only their belief and expectation in the power of an inert substance. About 93 percent of the patients who actually received antidepressant drugs experienced lessening of depressive symptoms—a higher proportion than those on the placebo. This result suggests that some patients are going to respond better to medications than they are to mind body interventions. Different treatments work in different ways with different people. But of course mind body interventions are often preferable, because drugs are accompanied by the risk of side effects such as addiction, by higher costs, and by other negative factors not associated with the placebo effect.

The research also raises intriguing possibilities for practical treatment techniques to alleviate depression through positive belief and expectation. A 2007 study published in *Behaviour Research and Therapy* evaluated the impact of five treatment interventions to treat depression in adolescents at high risk for this disorder, and also a "waitlist" control group that used no treatment.[15] The research showed that the waitlist controls received no benefits, while *all five of the active interventions* worked to significantly reduce depressive symptoms by the end of the study. The researchers concluded that a major component in the success of these interventions may have been the *expectancy* on the part of participants that the particular intervention they were involved in would work.

The five treatment interventions used by the investigators in this study included the following:

A cognitive behavioral therapy (CBT) depression prevention program. Typically, a CBT program will involve examining and adjusting negative assumptions about life (e.g., focusing on the positive aspects of a situation rather than only the negative aspects); keeping a diary of feelings, emotions, and behaviors; and learning to change one's typical, negative responses to stressful situations. Those involved in CBT therapies may also learn how to trigger the relaxation response and how to make use of distractions to get their minds off negative thoughts.

This approach resulted in superior success rates in treating depression, according to the evaluations of patients done by the researchers at follow-up points after the study was completed.

Supportive-expressive group intervention. Effective group therapy works extremely well in a variety of settings, including the various 12-step programs. Typically, group members focus at meetings on a particular problem shared by all participants (in this case, depression). They engage in open discussion of each person's feelings and emphasize the importance of positive, supportive responses.

Supportive and expressive group interventions may complement or overlap with CBT or other types of psychotherapeutic treatment. Like CBT, the supportive-expressive group intervention approach employed in this study provided a superior method for decreasing depressive symptoms, not only immediately after the prevention study but also at one- and six-month follow-up intervals.

Bibliotherapy. Bibliotherapy is based on the assumption that the simple act of reading can produce healing of various health conditions, including depression. The definition of bibliotherapy has broadened over the years to include using any type of reading material that is uplifting or emotionally sustaining. Patients may also employ other media that are similarly positive or salubrious, including videos and movies.

Therapeutic reading ranked toward the top of the interventions, along with CBT and supportive-expressive groups, as a highly effective method of decreasing depressive symptoms.

Expressive writing. Expressive writing includes writing about feelings or memories. Just putting a particular feeling—such as depression or anxiety—into words can lessen the effect of the emotion.

Journaling. Journaling is a form of expressive writing that emphasizes making regular entries in a diary or journal over an extended period of time. Journal writers typically record a variety of emotions over weeks or months. Journal writing can be similar to the expressive writing described above in that both types focus on objectifying and understanding high-stress, negative emotions.

A potential danger in journaling or any other type of expressive writing is that the writer may focus on negative emotions over extended periods. He or she may actually begin to wallow in those emotions rather than deal with them constructively. The result may be a kind of backfire effect, with the writing associated with a deepening of anxiety or depression.

In a 2005 study over a 12-week period, women with newly diagnosed breast cancer engaged in "expressive journaling" as a possible means to reduce stress. But they actually increased levels of anxiety and depression because of their excessive focus on negative emotions. The researchers concluded that their findings "suggest the need for additional research into the naturalistic application of journaling so that appropriate recommendations for writing (e.g., focus, timing, amount) can be offered to patients who might choose to utilize this approach for coping with the stresses of cancer diagnosis and treatment."[16]

This cautionary note should alert you as a patient, as well as your physician, to the importance of always keeping your ultimate objective in mind as you pursue any therapy designed to heal emotions. Your goal should be to develop a consistently *positive* mental picture of the state of good health that you want to achieve. An important part of the healing power of each of the activities mentioned above—CBT, supportive-expressive groups, bibliotherapy, expressive writing, and journaling—lies not primarily in the activities themselves. Rather, recovery depends on tapping into the power of inner conviction and anticipation that a particular therapeutic activity will actually lead to improvement of health. (For a detailed approach to treating depression using our two-phase Benson-Henry Protocol, see Chapter 7, page 123.)

The Placebo Effect and Parkinson's Disease

The classic Fuente-Fernández study[17] established the placebo effect as a powerful strategy to combat Parkinson's disease, which is characterized by the body's inadequate production of the neurotransmitter dopamine. Symptoms of Parkinson's disease include tremors, muscle rigidity, slow movement, poor balance, and a shuffling gait.

Typically, Parkinson's is treated by the medication levodopa (or L-dopa), which is converted by the body into dopamine. But in this study, the researchers employed the placebo effect by having the patients take inert pills rather than levodopa. Those receiving the placebo assumed that they were being treated by valid medications for their Parkinson's.

The researchers' surprising finding was the placebo pills actually caused the patients' bodies to produce levodopa. The healing factor was simply that the patients *believed* the inert pills would work. In some instances, the placebo worked better than the actual medication. Later studies and review articles have confirmed that when a researcher verbally induces expectations in a test subject that motor movement in Parkinson's disease *will* improve, the motor movement actually *does* improve.[18]

In a related experiment published in 2004 in the *Archives of General Psychiatry*,[19] researchers measured the responses to surgery between two groups of Parkinson's patients. The first group of patients received real surgery: a transplant of human tissue—specifically, embryonic dopamine neurons—into the brain. The second group received sham surgery: They were given surface burr incisions in the head, but no surgical entry into the brain. All participated in the experiment with full knowledge and consent that half of the group would not be given the real surgery but also with the understanding that those getting the sham incision could receive the actual surgical treatment later if the method worked to relieve Parkinson's symptoms.* Finally, this investigation was designed as a double-blind study, with neither patients nor researchers being aware of who was getting the real treatment and who was not.

The researchers found that those who *perceived* they had received the transplants—even if they hadn't—not only experienced increased levels of L-dopa but also reported better scores on various "quality of life" measurements, including improved physical symptoms related to Parkinson's. A major limitation of these studies is that the beneficial effects on Parkinson's patients have been observed only over relatively short time periods. The longer-term therapeutic value remains to be established in future studies. In any case, the patients' expectations or belief in improvement actually led to improvement.

These results demonstrate the tremendous power of the mind, through the mechanism of the belief system, to produce a natural neurotransmitter that had previously been deficient in the body. Still, the question of how to trigger such a response in the average patient presents an intriguing challenge. If a physician tells a patient that a placebo is a real medication, the patient may believe the doctor and improve. But such an approach places the doctor in the untenable situation of having to lie to the patient.

On the other hand, a physician trained in mind body strategies may help patients generate a belief that they can get well. If this personal belief grows sufficiently strong, the likelihood increases that patients in a doctor's office will have the same ability to improve as

---

* Although ethical objections have been raised to using sham surgery as a placebo, the practice continues to be employed on the grounds that this approach to scientific investigation meets U.S. federal regulations governing human-subject research. (See A. J. London, "Placebos That Harm: Sham Surgery Controls in Clinical Trials," *Statistical Methods in Medical Research,* Oct. 2002, 11(5): 413–27.)

patients in the Fuente-Fernández study. (For a detailed approach to treating Parkinson's disease using our two-phase Benson-Henry Protocol, see Chapter 7, page 176.)

So how can you and your doctor take advantage of this expectation-belief mechanism?

Many times, the evidence of this mechanism's healing power has emerged accidentally, as a by-product of the research protocols of modern science. The control group in a double-blind study will typically be given a placebo of some sort, such as an inert pill, a sham procedure, or a task that has no known health benefit. But in designing healing options that rely on the expectation-belief mechanism, physicians cannot ethically give a patient a dummy pill or treatment without informing the patient. Also, what patient would submit to a treatment known to be ineffective?

To meet these objections—and to move beyond them to the healing that is possible with mind body treatments—we recommend that you tap the power of your beliefs and expectations through the following steps:

- *Understand and accept with conviction* the efficacy of the scientific research in the realm of belief and expectation.

The scientific record is clear; your challenge is to accept it as fact. *Simply trusting in the facts* will take you most of the way toward appropriating the healing power of belief.

- *Expect* the scientific research to apply to you personally and to your particular disease or health complaint.

Suppose, for instance, that you are suffering from some form of chronic pain or depression. You know reputable studies have established that the mind has alleviated or cured a similar condition in others. Wouldn't it be reasonable for you to assume that if you can generate a similar level of belief, you will be likely to trigger your innate ability to overcome pain or depression?

- Develop a *consistent and systematic treatment strategy* to apply what you know and believe to your practical situation.

To help you achieve your goal of good health, we have established a set of proven steps and procedures in Part II, which describe in practical detail how you can incorporate both the relaxation response and healing expectation-belief into your personal health plan.

Part II

Designing Your Personal Mind Body Treatment Plan

6.

Planning Your Personal Mind Body Health Strategy

Peter had been diagnosed with hypertension, with readings that often spiked to dangerously high levels. His condition, which is a problem for more than an estimated 60 million Americans, was of particular concern because high blood pressure put him at risk for a number of serious health problems, including strokes, heart attacks, and kidney failure.

Even though Peter was taking antihypertensive medications, his measurements typically were in the 158/88 mm Hg range. Normal blood pressure guidelines, according to the National Heart, Lung, and Blood Institute, should be below 120/80. The "prehypertension" levels—that is, the levels at which a person is at higher-than-normal risk for hypertension—range from 120/80 to 139/89. Any readings for either the systolic (upper) or diastolic (lower) number above 140/90 are considered hypertension. Peter was well into the systolic hypertension range and was close to having diastolic hypertension.

As for exactly what caused his hypertension, there were telltale danger signals. For one thing, he reported to me that his job was highly stressful. Also, Peter said that he often responded to stressful situations with anger and frustration, and had a great deal of difficulty controlling these negative emotions. Furthermore, I knew from his patient history that hypertension ran in his family: His father had suffered from the condition before dying of a stroke.

Learning that Peter was a Roman Catholic who attended church regularly, I decided to help him design a mind body treatment that took advantage of his faith. First, I asked him to remember what it felt like to worship and pray in church.

"That's frequently my only moment of peace during the week," he said.

With that information in mind, I taught Peter a simple, standard technique for evoking the relaxation response by using a short prayer of his choosing, which he repeated silently over and over.* I asked him to remember his feelings and his environment while he was praying in church. In effect, he moved from an elicitation of the relaxation response to a visualization of what it felt like to be stress free in the most peaceful surroundings that he could remember.

When I saw Peter several months later, his blood pressure had declined to 124/72. Also, he reported that he was feeling much calmer and more in control of his emotions. He was continuing with his previous medication program but was now experiencing almost normal pressure. If he had failed to bring the pressure readings down, he would have been forced to increase the dose of the drug.

Peter's experience introduces a practical treatment approach that serves as a paradigm for the practical applications of mind body science. Sometimes, this mind body healing protocol works so well that drugs or other medical interventions are unnecessary. Other times, as in Peter's situation, a *combination treatment* may be best: a mind body approach *plus* drugs or surgery.

The basic two-part Benson-Henry Protocol,† which Peter followed, can be summarized this way:

---

* For a detailed description of the technique, see page 93.
† The two-phase Benson-Henry Protocol introduced here shares a common base with the Relaxation Response Resiliency Enhancement Programs that are offered by our Institute.

Phase One: Relaxation Response Trigger. This basic template, which requires 12 to 15 minutes and should be used for *all* mind body treatments, will, by itself, trigger a number of beneficial physiologic and genetic expression changes in your body. Then, move on to Phase Two.

Phase Two: Visualization. This second component of effective mind body treatment usually requires 8 to 10 minutes and has been tailored in Chapter 7 to deal with a wide variety of health problems. The visualization exercise is designed to enhance healing through memories that will reinforce your expectations and beliefs.

We have included boxes summarizing this two-phase protocol in Chapter 1, page 9, and also in Chapter 7, page 111. In the following sections, however, we go into Phase One and Phase Two in more detail so that you will have all the information you should need to understand each phase fully and to design your own treatment program most effectively.

Phase One: Relaxation Response Trigger

Your objective in Phase One is to create the distinctive physiologic and genetic conditions associated with the relaxation response.* These include such anti-stress changes as a healthier metabolism, lower blood pressure, slower heart and breathing rates, an overall calming of the brain, and a sense of relaxation and well-being. When these changes occur, you can assume that the beneficial changes in gene expression are also taking place.

How can you bring about these basic physiologic and genetic changes? You should start with Phase One of our Benson-Henry Protocol, which features the eight-step elicitation of the relaxation response.

---

* See Chapters 2 and 4.

Eight Steps to the Relaxation Response

Although many approaches will trigger the relaxation response in your body, for decades at the Harvard Medical School we have used—and proven scientifically—the following eight-step sequence:

Step 1: *Pick a focus word, phrase, image, or short prayer* for your relaxation response session. Or choose just to focus on your breathing.

Any word or phrase with neutral or positive connotations—such as *one* or *peace*—will be fine for this purpose. Just remember that if you choose only one word, you should draw it out during your entire exhaled breath as you silently repeat it.

If possible, the word, phrase, or prayer you select should be emotionally soothing and should conform to your deepest beliefs or worldview. For example, a Christian might pick *Lord Jesus*; a Jew, *Echod*; a Hindu or Buddhist, *Om*; or a Muslim, *Insha'Allah*.

There is a twofold reason for these criteria: First, it is easier to form and reinforce a positive habit if you are repeating words that you believe in. Second, expectation or belief that a technique will work in our mind and body is more likely to cause that technique to work.

Step 2: *Find a quiet place* where you are unlikely to be interrupted, and sit calmly in a comfortable position.

Step 3: *Close your eyes.*

Step 4: *Progressively relax all your muscles,* beginning with your toes and feet and moving up through your entire body, shoulders, and face. Spend a minute or two with this relaxation exercise.

Step 5: *Breathe slowly and naturally.* As you exhale, repeat silently your focus word, phrase, or prayer, or picture the image you have chosen. Or focus on your breathing rhythm, if you have chosen a breath focus for this exercise.

Step 6: *Assume a passive attitude* throughout the session. Don't worry about how you are doing; you can be sure that just by following these eight steps, you are changing your physiology from a stress response to the relaxation response.

When other thoughts come to your mind—as they are sure to

do—simply think, "Oh well," and turn away from the distraction and back to your focus word, phrase, prayer, or breathing. Do not become concerned if you notice that your particular health symptoms, such as a headache or other pain, briefly intensify during your first few sessions. This reaction is normal, because as your mind becomes more sensitized and focused, your aches and pains may naturally come to the fore.

Step 7: *Continue with this exercise for 12 to 15 minutes.* The average time for most beginning patients to achieve the maximum health benefits from this Phase One treatment is within this range. After a patient has practiced this procedure for several weeks, the health benefits can often be achieved more quickly, though we still recommend that patients keep 12 to 15 minutes as their treatment goal for each session.

Step 8: *Practice this technique at least once daily,* preferably in the morning before breakfast or in the afternoon or early evening just before dinner. Make a commitment to this daily practice for at least 30 consecutive days, which is approximately the time necessary for a new habit to be established.[1]

But our eight-step sequence is only one approach that you may use to evoke the relaxation response. Countless other ways are also available for entering this healing physiologic state, provided you observe several simple guidelines.

Other Relaxation Response Exercises

Additional activities may also produce the relaxation response. Simply incorporate three essential components into your chosen activity:*

1. *A mental focusing device* that will help you break the pattern of everyday thoughts and concerns. The device can involve words, images, or physical actions such as breathing or footsteps.

---

* You will note that all three of these components are mentioned in the above eight-step standard relaxation response exercise.

2. *A passive, "oh well" attitude* toward distracting thoughts. If distracting thoughts, including everyday worries or concerns, take over your mind during the exercise, the physiologic effects of the relaxation response may not occur.

3. *Sufficient time*—at least 12 to 15 consecutive minutes per practice session—to allow the requisite physiologic changes to occur.

Here are a few suggestions—by no means an exhaustive list!—about ways to generate the relaxation response on your own, apart from the standard eight-step exercise:

Repetitive aerobic exercise. Walking, jogging, cycling, or swimming can produce the effect, provided you are in good enough physical condition to continue the activity for at least 12 to 15 minutes without becoming anaerobic, or short of breath. Exercises that require a short burst of high energy or that require great concentration on playmaking, such as tennis or basketball, are not as conducive to producing the relaxation response.

Eastern meditative exercises. You may already be engaging in such practices as yoga, tai chi, Qigong, Transcendental Meditation, or mindfulness meditation. These are all examples of effective relaxation response exercises, which have philosophical roots in Eastern religions.

But with these techniques, remember that scientific studies have established that the anti-stress physiologic response—the relaxation response—does *not* depend primarily on any particular belief system. Rather, the capacity to experience the relaxation response is biologically innate, built into every human mind and body and accessible to all by the appropriate techniques.

Repetitive prayer. In Western religions, repeating words, phrases, or longer passages from a familiar liturgical prayer, the Bible, or another sacred text can produce the relaxation response. Your selection may be repeated in the context of a familiar and comforting practice or ritual, rather than used as part of our standard eight-step approach.

An important aspect of using a repetitive prayer from your faith tradition is to assume that "God is on my side in this endeavor. God has made me with this innate healing capacity, and He wants me to make the best use of it." Make it clear to yourself that you possess a positive belief in the power of the mind body exercise to heal. As a means of enhancing your belief, it is often helpful to remind yourself that you really do believe in the particular repetitive prayer you are using.

Here are a few examples of the kinds of repetitive prayer that are typically rooted in deep personal belief:

"Hail Mary, full of grace."
"The Lord is One."
"The Lord is my shepherd."
"Lord have mercy."
"The peace of God."
"Insha'Allah."

Progressive muscle relaxation. Progressive muscle relaxation, which is featured in Step 4 of our eight-step sequence, can also be used by itself to achieve the desired results. Just focus during the entire 12-to-15-minute session on relaxing different muscles and muscle groups throughout your body and also on your own steady breathing.

Playing a musical instrument or singing. Some find that playing memorized sequences on an instrument can trigger the relaxation response. Others may prefer chanting or singing.

Listening to music. Soothing music—either instrumental or voice-based with chanting or familiar, repetitive phrases—can be effective in achieving the desired physiologic responses. But music that is loud, cacophonous, or otherwise nonrestful tends to work against the desired healing effect.

Engaging in a task that requires "mindless" repetitive movements. Such activities may involve gardening, tinkering on a machine such as an auto, woodworking, knitting, or doing needlepoint.

"Natural" triggers. People have reported the relaxation response experience after lengthy, quiet exposure to water, such as floating in a calm pool; lying for a similar length of time in a full, relaxing bathtub; or simply standing under a shower.

Others have the relaxation response experience while sitting alone in the woods and contemplating natural sights; lying on their back and looking up at the sky; or sitting by the ocean and watching and listening to the steady drumbeat of the waves.

The Olivia CD. As you know from Chapter 2, a specially designed audio recording called the "Olivia CD" has been used with great success in many of our scientific experiments at the Harvard Medical School.[*]

All the techniques described above can be utilized by anyone without any special equipment, other than a simple CD player. A number of studies have also shown that the relaxation response can be elicited by using sophisticated equipment, such as biofeedback machines, or by approaches such as hypnosis that require trained medical personnel. But our main focus is on those techniques that can be employed by individual patients on their own, after they have received simple instruction through this book or from qualified instructors.

As with our eight-step relaxation response procedure, the options summarized above should be practiced at least once daily for an average of 12 to 15 minutes each session. Also, be sure to incorporate the three basic principles mentioned earlier in this chapter on page 95: 1) a consistent mental focus; 2) a passive attitude toward distractions; and 3) sufficient time for each session.

Measuring Your Success in Eliciting the Relaxation Response
How can you be sure that the approach you have chosen is actually

---

[*] See a more detailed description of the Olivia CD on page 24. If you are interested in ordering the CD, which is titled *Bring Relaxation to Your Life* by Olivia Hoblitzelle, please visit our website, www.massgeneral.org/bhi, and click on the link to the "Online Store."

working—and enhancing your innate healing potential? Here are several helpful tests:

- If you feel more relaxed after you finish a Phase One session, the technique is working.
- If the symptoms you experience diminish or disappear, even momentarily, during or immediately after a session, the technique is working.
- If the symptoms you experience diminish within a week or two, the technique is working.
- If you feel that the stressors in your life bother you less now than they did when you started this mind body treatment process, the technique is working.
- If you feel that you are more in control of your life now than when you started, the technique is working.
- If you are observing the basic guidelines for eliciting the relaxation response, you can rest assured, in light of the extensive scientific studies, that the technique is working—no matter how you may feel on a day-to-day basis.

But evoking the relaxation response is just the first phase in an effective mind body treatment strategy. Phase Two will provide enhanced potential for healing.

Phase Two: Visualization

Experiencing Phase One on a regular basis—that is, simply evoking the relaxation response daily—will often lead to significant healing without any further action. But you will increase your chances for maximum healing by adding Phase Two—the visualization phase—to your mind body medicine kit.

In Phase Two, you will continue to intensify your Phase One relaxation response experience by focusing on calming, soothing memories or other mental imagery. Typically, these memories and images will be linked to your belief system.

So how does Phase Two work? The answer requires an understanding of mental visualization.*

How Visualization Works

When you have finished a relaxation response session after 12 to 15 minutes, you are ready to move from Phase One to Phase Two of the Benson-Henry Protocol. Your brain is now calmer, more focused, and more open to healthful suggestions and information.† In this mental state, you are physiologically prepared to follow a visualization procedure that can enhance the healing process.

The Phase Two Procedure

Sit quietly with your eyes closed and picture what it was like to be free of the disease or symptom that you are experiencing. If your problem is back pain, for instance, you might remember yourself as a younger person, moving, walking, twisting your upper body, or jogging easily, with no discomfort. This mental exercise will help you *remember* and even *relive a state of wellness* that you enjoyed in the past.

If you can't recall a time when you were symptom free, just visualize what you *think* or *imagine* it would be like to move about without the pain. Or if you have trouble forming mental images, focus on your body *right now*, in your present circumstances. Imagine you are standing up and then moving easily and smoothly to the other side of the room, or climbing up and down a nearby flight of stairs, or performing some other physical act—but without any pain or discomfort.

Picture yourself engaging in any physical act that you would like to be able to do without pain or other symptoms. You might see yourself throwing a ball, swinging a tennis racket, gardening, play-

---

* See Chapter 5, page 72, for the scientific foundation for healing through expectation and belief.

† For a discussion of the scientific basis for these brain changes—i.e., *why* visualization works—see the following section in this chapter.

ing some pickup basketball, or kicking a soccer ball with a child or grandchild. Your choice of mental picture should be personal; select an activity that you enjoy doing but have found you can't do because of your symptoms. The main idea in Phase Two is to identify your particular symptom or disease, but then to see yourself completely healed of that symptom or disease.

Hold these dynamic inner images in your mind for 8 to 10 minutes and play with them in your imagination. Construct a kind of mental motion picture where you are the healthy central character.

After the 8-to-10-minute period, continue to sit quietly for about a minute with your eyes closed, but this time, allow "regular" thoughts to reenter your mind. Then open your eyes and continue sitting quietly for about another minute. Finally, return to your normal activities.

Continue Applying the Basic Principles

Many of the basic principles you learned in the Phase One exercise continue to apply in Phase Two. For example, maintaining a passive attitude remains important. So if you find your mind wanders as you visualize yourself in a completely healthy state, don't fight the distractions. Just say silently, "Oh well," and return gently to your mental picture.

Also, you may find that during the visualization your symptoms, such as pain, intensify. Just continue with the protocol, and expect that soon these symptoms will ease.

The Performance Paradox

A paradox that appears with many of my patients is that even though they are supposed to become more relaxed and stress free during Phase Two, at the outset they begin to worry, "Am I doing this right? Is my visualization technique really okay? Should I be dwelling on some different memory from the one I've chosen?"

Here is a typical, simple response that I give to such performance-focused anxieties:

"Don't worry about how well you're doing! Don't worry about whether the relaxation response is really working or whether your mental picture is maximizing your health benefits. Just do it!"

I also frequently use the analogy of brushing teeth. Most of us are concerned to one extent or another with dental hygiene, but we don't dwell on the tooth-cleaning process. We just work away with that brush every day. Almost no one evaluates the brushing, to say, "That was a good brush!" or, "Too bad—that was a bad brush." We simply do it!

Similarly, if you're taking a pill your doctor has prescribed for your cholesterol or blood pressure, you probably don't wonder, "Am I putting this pill in the proper side of my mouth? Am I swallowing it correctly? Is it really going to work?" Again, you just do it—and that should be your approach to mind body treatments.

Just practice Phases One and Two and avoid evaluating your performance or cataloging changes in your body or emotions. Beneficial changes usually occur over time. And as you experience some relief, your confidence will grow that mind body healing is working—just as brushing and flossing teeth or taking appropriately prescribed pills works. By developing healthy mind body habits, you will continue to build upon your positive expectations that the treatment will be effective. At the same time, you will increasingly turn away from any opposite, unhealthy focus, which may involve remembering the state and symptoms of *illness* rather than remembering what it was like, or could be like, to *be well.*

Why exactly does visualization work? Some interesting scientific research may point us toward possible answers.

Why Does Visualization Work?

Two important areas of scientific thinking can help explain the validity of the visualization techniques advocated in this book: 1) our research into the calming and focusing of the brain, and 2) the role of memory in helping patients access the power of belief and expectation in mind body treatments.

Calming and Focusing the Brain

The two-phase protocol we have established for mind body healing is designed to conform to brain research in this way: *Starting* a treatment with the Phase One relaxation response trigger will calm the mind and maximize the healing impact of Phase Two visualization.

In a study conducted at the Massachusetts General Hospital under the leadership of Sara W. Lazar and published in *NeuroReport* in 2000, we used functional magnetic resonance imaging (fMRI) to identify brain regions that were active during a simple form of meditation that evoked the relaxation response.[2] The subjects were long-time experts in this Phase One meditation technique, which involved repeating one short phrase on the out-breath and another phrase on the in-breath.*

We concluded from this experiment that the repetitive mental technique for eliciting the relaxation response had caused beneficial changes in the attention and executive control parts of the subjects' brains. Overall, the "static" in the brain, including thoughts and worries that may interfere with concentration, decreased as the subjects continued with their mental exercise. Their brains tended to become calmer and more open to new thoughts. The computerized fMRI pictures, through highlighted images, showed decreased and more focused brain activity.

What are the benefits of these findings for Phase Two of our Benson-Henry Protocol?

First, the brain changes in Phase One prepare patients to visualize more clearly and calmly in Phase Two a state of being free from medical symptoms, such as pain or other discomforts. Also, their minds become more open to forgetting ingrained symptoms and incorporating healing beliefs and expectations. Finally, their bodies are freer of the stress responses that cause or exacerbate illness.

But this calming and focusing of the brain is only one of the fac-

---

* We have described this study in some detail, but in another context and with a different purpose, in our previous book, *The Breakout Principle* (New York: Scribner, 2003, 2004), 71ff.

tors that give the visualization component of the protocol its power. Another factor involves a special type of memory.

The Power of Memory

To help patients access their full potential to be healed through expectation and belief, I have developed a memory-related concept that encompasses, but also moves beyond, the healing power of the placebo effect. This concept, which I have introduced in the medical literature, is called "remembered wellness." My research and clinical practice in recent years have confirmed my earlier conclusions about remembered wellness. We have also found that the placebo effect works on many more symptoms and illnesses than we first thought.

What is remembered wellness?

As already indicated in Chapter 1 on pages 13 and 14, this term refers to the utilization in the healing process of one or more memories of a past state of wellness.[3] Typically, these memories can be accessed and employed for medical treatment through a process of visualization, or the use of mental images and pictures, which may be built around actual memories of being healthy, strong, and resilient.

A simple illustration of how remembered wellness works was brought home to me at a lecture I delivered to physicians and scientists at the Semel Institute, UCLA. After explaining the science that undergirds the phenomenon, I led the audience through a brief session where I had them evoke the relaxation response themselves. Then, after I had fielded some questions and ended my presentation, several people approached me with further questions, including a smiling elderly man.

To my surprise I learned that the man was 92, much older than he looked. He was also an internationally known, widely published physicist. But the important part of the story for our purposes involved what had happened to him when, as a member of the audience, he had evoked the relaxation response for the first time:

"I had these wonderful feelings of being young again!" he said.

He revealed that his focus for the exercise had been a Jewish prayer, which he had often used during his youth.

"When I was quite young, I had to make a decision about whether to become a physicist or a rabbi," he said. "I loved the idea of rabbinical studies and wished that I could follow both paths. But I had to make a choice. Today, when I used that prayer from my youth, I felt young again."

For a few moments, this man had relived the invigorating memories of a happy earlier stage of his life. In the process, he had broken the train of everyday thought and put aside for a short time the stresses of living. Subjectively, his personal observations suggest an enhanced state of wellness. From a more objective medical point of view, we can say that his mind—specifically his memories of a vital youth—had provided his body with new energy. From what we know about the biological changes that accompany such an experience, we can be reasonably certain that his body had alleviated the effects of stressful hormones, such as norepinephrine; fMRI readings would have shown a calmer brain; and his gene expression had even changed for the better.

In short, he had undergone a fleeting experience of remembered wellness.

Remembered wellness versus the placebo effect

Remembered wellness differs significantly from the placebo effect, at least as that concept has evolved in modern medical understanding. For one thing, the placebo effect typically occurs without the patient's volition or knowledge—and may even be evoked through deception or trickery. For example, as we have already seen, a physician may give an inert pill to a patient yet tell the patient that it contains a real medication designed to help with a particular medical problem. Remembered wellness, in contrast, occurs when the patient, in full knowledge of the need to believe or expect positive results, *wills* the belief and expectation to occur.[4]

Another difference from the placebo effect is that remembered

---

105

wellness is based on a positive, *wellness-based medical model* rather than on the typical *disease-based model* followed by most physicians and researchers. The main use of the placebo effect in recent years has been with control groups in experiments that are testing the effect of various drugs on certain diseases. If a placebo-using group does as well medically as a drug-using group, then the drug is usually deemed ineffective in treating the disease. But the effect of the placebo, which is sometimes greater than that of the drug, is usually ignored.

A third reason that remembered wellness is different from the placebo effect is that, as the name implies, remembered wellness is rooted in the patient's *memories of good health*. These recollections may arise from the patient's actual experiences of being symptom free, or they may be associated mainly with the patient's ideas of what complete good health and wellness might be like.

No clinical details—no bad memories!
When you draw mental pictures during Phase Two visualization, avoid picturing meticulous medical procedures, biological processes, or some "get-well-quick" self-help system. The more you focus on your specific medical problem, the less powerful your visualization will become. Even a fleeting memory of unpleasant symptoms, such as pain, may overstimulate pain centers in the brain and cause pain to intensify. This process causes "phantom pain" in missing limbs. That is, if you lose an arm or a leg, at times you might actually feel pain in that limb—even though the limb no longer exists.

Healing Through Cognitive Behavioral Therapy (CBT)
Cognitive behavioral therapy refers, in general, to healing methods designed to change destructive or unhealthful emotions that may also have an unhealthy effect on your body.* If you expect to be depressed, or to feel pain, or to be fearful, your negative expectations have a good

---

* See Chapter 5, page 83.

chance of becoming reality. But if you can somehow transform your thinking into a more positive mindset, your mind can influence your body and emotions in a happier, calmer, healthier direction. Two important ways in which Phase Two visualization may make use of CBT are cognitive restructuring and desensitization.

Rebuilding Your Mental Reactions Through Cognitive Restructuring
Cognitive restructuring, which can change negative emotions that harm health, may be employed in Phase Two when you visualize or remember a healthful state that is the polar opposite of your illness.

Suppose that you suffer from lower-back pain, which prevents you from engaging in activities you enjoy. But now, after you have experienced the relaxation response and opened your mind in Phase One, you might construct a mental picture of yourself engaging in those previous activities, but without pain. By visualizing a strong back over many days as part of your mind body treatment, you will gradually replace your expectation of pain with an expectation of a healed back. You will in effect *condition* your mind to expect health and *decondition* your mind to expect illness.

Many of the visualizations we suggest in the next chapter are based on this assumption: *You can restructure your thinking processes to expect good health rather than bad.* With that expectation, your mind will more likely influence your body in a healthful direction.

Desensitization
At times in Phase Two, we will suggest that you employ visualization to desensitize yourself to unhealthful thoughts or emotional responses. The main idea is that by exposing yourself to the condition or object that you suffer from or fear, you become less sensitive and vulnerable to that condition or fear.

This approach can be especially useful in treating phobias and various forms of anxiety that are connected with a particular feared situation or object. For example, if you "turn to putty" emotionally when you have to give a speech or take a test, exposure to the feared challenge through mental imagery over a period of time can reduce the intensity of the negative emotions considerably.

With this Benson-Henry Protocol in mind—the Phase One relaxation response trigger and the Phase Two visualization—you are now ready to explore specific mind body treatments for specific illnesses or medical conditions. This basic "mind body medical kit" should provide you with what you need to maximize your inherent healing potential.

7.

A Guide to Specific Mind Body Treatments

Some patients have asked, "I have several family health guides at home—but why isn't there a *Family Mind Body Health Guide*?" This part of the book fills that gap. The following pages contain a practical, stand-alone medical guide to proven mind body techniques that can be used to treat dozens of specific diseases and health conditions.

In some cases, the mind body treatment alone is sufficient to deal with a medical problem. In others, you and your physician will find it advisable to use the mind body approaches described in this section *in combination with* standard medical treatments, such as drugs and surgery. By using this combination treatment, you may find that you can reduce your medication dosage or have less invasive surgical procedures.

The mind body model we recommend—which has already been introduced in Chapter 1 on page 18, and which should be part of any overall treatment scheme—can be summarized this way.

Step 1: Symptoms
With your doctor's guidance, identify your medical symptoms and specific diagnosis. Inform your physician about your intention to

employ a mind body approach in your treatment plan. To select an appropriate mind body approach, ask your doctor to help interpret your medical diagnosis and symptoms. Sometimes, as with conditions such as hypertension, you may not be experiencing any telltale symptoms, but diagnostic procedures will reveal that you do have a problem.

Step 2: Standard Medical Treatments
Again with your physician's guidance, evaluate the standard medical treatments for your condition, including drugs or surgery. Your physician will help you understand possible side effects of medications and also the likelihood of improvement or cure with drugs and/or surgery.

Step 3: Scientific Proof for Mind Body Approaches
Next, explore your third medical option—a mind body treatment. This step is particularly important if there is a stress component in your complaint.

Step 4: Possible Mind Body Treatments
If you and your physician determine that a mind body approach should be applied to relieve your condition, you should proceed with our two-phase Benson-Henry Protocol. This protocol includes the Phase One relaxation response trigger, an exercise that will take about 12 to 15 minutes.

Then spend about 8 to 10 minutes engaging in Phase Two visualization, which will engage the healing power of expectation, belief, and memory. Practice the visualization protocol immediately after you elicit the relaxation response, because at that point your mind is most open to new learning and healthful conditioning. The total amount of time for the entire two-phase protocol will be 20 to 25 minutes each day.

The specific mind body treatments for dozens of medical conditions described in the following pages have been designed to conform to this model. You will see that we have included examples of particular types of visualization that clinical practice has suggested may work well with particular types of medical conditions. But you should feel free to vary your visualization, depending on the particular mental picture that may reinforce your expectation-belief in the possibility of successful treatment.

You will note that we have designed the format so that you can use this chapter as a self-contained medical reference guide. If you are suffering from a particular medical condition, you may choose to consult only the description of and recommendations for that condition. In this way, you will have access to a stand-alone mind body treatment plan for an illness or medical condition you may encounter. For ease of reference, we have included a summary of the two-phase Benson-Henry Protocol* in the accompanying box (another summary can be found in the box in Chapter 1, page 9). When you arrive at the "Possible Mind Body Treatments" section of a given disease and prepare to embark on a treatment, you will be referred back to this summary as a guide to help you move through Phases One and Two of the protocol.

The Benson-Henry Protocol

Total time required daily for the protocol is **20 to 25 minutes,** allotted as follows:

PHASE ONE: Relaxation Response Trigger

Step 1: Focus on a word, phrase, image, short prayer, or your breathing.
Step 2: Find a quiet place and sit calmly in a comfortable position.
Step 3: Close your eyes.
Step 4: Progressively relax all your muscles.

---

* The two-phase Benson-Henry Protocol introduced here shares a common base with the Relaxation Response Resiliency Enhancement Programs that are offered by our Institute.

Step 5: Breathe slowly and naturally. As you exhale, concentrate on your focus.

Step 6: Assume a passive attitude. When thoughts intrude, simply think, "Oh well," and return to your focus.

Step 7: Continue this exercise for an average of 12 to 15 minutes.

Step 8: Practice this technique at least once daily.

Option: Use one of the optional relaxation response exercises described on page 95, but remember to incorporate three essential components:

1. *A mental focusing device to break the pattern of everyday thoughts.*
2. *A passive, "oh well" attitude toward distracting thoughts.*
3. *Sufficient time—an average of 12 to 15 consecutive minutes.*

Important: To ensure genetic effects, practice Phase One daily for at least eight weeks. For the maximal genetic effect as established by our research, the exercise should be practiced for many years.

PHASE TWO: Visualization

Visualize for 8 to 10 minutes to engage expectation, belief, and memory.

Angina Pectoris (Chest Pain Caused by Heart Disease)

Symptoms

Chest pains can result from a variety of conditions, such as a heart attack, muscle tension, reflux from the stomach into the esophagus, or even shingles. But the specific chest pain known as *angina* or *angina pectoris*—literally translated from the Latin as "strangling of the chest"—is most often caused by blockage of the coronary arteries. The blocks result from the buildup of plaque and blood clots in those arteries. The decreased flow of blood into the heart produces a condition known as *ischemia,* or lack of adequate oxygen to the muscles of the heart. As less blood and oxygen reach these muscles, the patient may feel pressure, heaviness, burning, or aching in the chest, arms, or shoulders, especially just after the "three E's": exercise, emotion, and eating.[1] Each "E" requires more blood flow to the heart to deliver more oxygen and without such blood flow, chest pain results.

Standard Medical Procedures and Treatments

Diagnostic procedures that can identify coronary artery blockage that may cause anginal pains include:

- the resting electrocardiogram (ECG), which involves placing several electrodes on the chest to monitor the heart's electrical action;
- the stress test, or exercise ECG (which also involves placing several electrodes on the chest, but this time to monitor the heart's electrical responses during vigorous exercise, usually on a treadmill or stationary bike);
- the injection and measurement of radioactive solutions, which move through the bloodstream into the heart during a stress test;
- an echocardiogram, or picturing the pumping of the heart by the use of ultrasound waves; and
- an arteriogram, or insertion of a dye into the coronary arteries to make it easier to view blockage (or occlusion) of the arteries through use of an X-ray.

If one or more of these tests reveal that the patient has coronary artery disease, several options are available for treatment of anginal pains. One is rest. Another is taking nitroglycerin. Also, lifestyle measures, including exercise, weight loss, stopping smoking, and stress management, often prove effective. More serious blockage may be treated by drugs, such as beta-blockers. Very serious or near-complete blockage of arteries may require surgery, such as a coronary artery bypass.

Scientific Proof for Mind Body Approaches

The power of mind body treatments to relieve angina pectoris has been reinforced in a number of scientific studies during the last three decades. As mentioned previously, David P. McCallie, Jr., and I, while at Boston's Beth Israel Hospital, concluded in a *New England Journal of Medicine* review that the placebo effect can reduce angina pains.[2]

We analyzed data from studies involving more than 1,000 patients who had used five different *inactive* treatments. These five placebo treatments included ineffectual drug therapies and useless surgical procedures, such as ligation, or tying off, of one of the small arteries inside the chest.

At first, these inert substances and surgeries, which both patients and physicians believed would work, reduced anginal pain in 70 to 90 percent of patients. But later, when the physicians began to question or disbelieve the efficacy of the treatments, the effectiveness rate decreased to 30 to 40 percent. *Strong belief by the physician applying the treatments* led to significant relief from anginal pains, while a physician's disbelief greatly reduced the patient's relief from the pain.

This phenomenon—the importance of the caregiver's belief—demonstrates the broad reach of the placebo effect. As you know from the definition of the placebo effect (pages 45–48) that has evolved in our research over the years, the placebo works most powerfully when there is a threefold belief: belief of the patient, belief of the caregiver, and a shared belief that results from the trust relationship between the patient and the physician.

In a 1999 German study,[3] researchers affirmed that with angina pectoris and various other medical conditions, "Treatment with placebo is frequently effective and cannot therefore be considered as 'non-treatment.'" Specifically, they found that in patients with angina pectoris, placebos produced a 10 percent increase in exercise tolerance—i.e., an increase in the treadmill walking time that was needed to trigger the onset of angina attacks and abnormal ECG readings.

The Role of the Relaxation Response

The placebo effect is not the only mind body factor that has relieved symptoms of angina; the relaxation response may also come into play.

In a 2005 report in the *European Journal of Cardiovascular Prevention and Rehabilitation,* researchers evaluated the effects of relaxation therapy on the recovery of patients from a heart attack and on prevention of a cardiac ischemic event.[4] Of the 27 studies they reviewed, they found that when patients were given "full relaxation therapy" (defined as at least nine hours of supervised instruction and discussion), several benefits ensued: The frequency of angina pectoris was reduced, irregular heartbeats and exercise-induced ischemia were reduced, and work attendance improved. Also, cardiac events occurred less frequently, and there were fewer cardiac deaths.

The researchers concluded that intensive, supervised relaxation practice enhances recovery from a cardiac event stemming from too little oxygen to the heart. They emphasized that relaxation practice is an important ingredient of cardiac rehabilitation, in addition to exercise and psychological education.

Possible Mind Body Treatments

Now, proceed through the two-phase Benson-Henry Protocol summarized on page 111. As you employ this protocol, consider the following uses and variations.

Aborting an Anginal Attack

You might overcome an attack through a "mini" exercise: At the beginning of the attack, take a deep breath and hold it for 10 seconds. Then exhale slowly and silently repeat your focus word, phrase, or prayer.

This exercise could abort the anginal attack, as it undercuts the power of one "E": negative, stressful emotions. The approach will be all the more successful if you have been regularly eliciting the relaxation response and your mind and body have been adequately conditioned. If this mini doesn't work, proceed with your standard, physician-approved medical treatments for angina, such as taking nitroglycerin.

Note: The application of the "mini" relaxation response exercise is not limited to problems with angina pectoris. Patients with *any* medical problem—or those who want to *prevent* a problem—should consider employing this short, 10-to-15-second version of Phase One at appropriate times during the day, especially when stress intensifies. (See the accompanying box for a summary of the "mini" technique.) We have designed the "mini" to be used *in addition to,* but *not in place of,* your regular Phase One relaxation response trigger. Doing your regular daily practice sessions of the two-phase protocol will reinforce the "mini," making it more likely that your stress levels will be reduced and the healing effects of the relaxation response will take hold.

The "Mini" Relaxation Response Technique

* Take a deep breath and hold it for about 7 to 10 seconds.
* Exhale completely, and as you do so, silently repeat your focus word or phrase.
* This entire procedure should take no more than 10 to 15 seconds.
* Continue to breathe regularly, and proceed with your normal activities.

Visualization for Angina Pectoris

Avoid any attempt to visualize the anginal pain itself. A positive visualization should always be used with no attempt to deal with the specific pain.

Here is an illustration of how the treatment procedure might work:
First, evoke the Phase One relaxation response for 12 to 15 minutes.

Next, move into Phase Two for 8 to 10 minutes. Construct a mental picture of yourself conducting an activity that would normally evoke an anginal attack, but this time, see yourself functioning *without* the pain. For example, you may have found in the past that walking three blocks, climbing stairs, an argument with a colleague at work, or even the stress of watching your child play a tennis match has triggered your anginal pain. But now, see yourself doing one or more of these stressful activities—minus the pain. To reinforce the painless nature of the exercise, you might imagine yourself smiling and breathing easily during the scene, with an overriding sense of inner peace and confidence.

Distracting thoughts or even anginal pain will almost certainly intrude at times as you enjoy this mental scene, but don't allow such distractions to sidetrack you from the mind body exercise. Just say, "Oh well," and return to a contemplation of your mental imagery.

Finally, be sure to inform your cardiologist about your intention to use the stress-reducing mind body treatments in this book. Keep your doctor apprised of every step you take to counter angina or other heart-related problems.

Anxiety

Symptoms

Anxiety refers to a group of emotions that may include a specific fear of an actual event in progress (such as giving a speech); a generalized sense of worry that may be hard or impossible to link to a particular cause; or some uncertainty about the future, even if it is unlikely that the feared event will occur.

Anxiety can encompass a wide range of symptoms.[5] Those who suffer from what is often called *performance anxiety* may "tighten up" at the prospect of having to take a test, give a speech, or perform some other public act on which they expect to be judged. They may experience shortness of breath; shaky hands or voice, perhaps including an inability to "get the words out"; copious perspiration; rapid heart rate; pounding of the heart (palpitations); or an inability to focus the mind on the task at hand. A musician giving a recital, for instance, may suddenly "go blank" before an audience and completely forget notes that have been memorized.

Some types of anxiety are harder to analyze. *Generalized anxiety disorder,* or a "free-floating anxiety," for instance, cannot be linked to a specific event or source but still causes the person to experience increased irritability and restlessness. Physical symptoms may include rapid breathing, hyperventilation (a sense of lacking adequate oxygen intake in the lungs), or gastrointestinal problems, such as queasiness or diarrhea.

An anxiety attack may become more severe, in the form of a *panic attack* or *panic disorder.* Symptoms may include the above anxiety symptoms but the physical manifestations are usually more pronounced, with feelings of choking or even dying.

Related problems may include various *phobias,* which are covered in a separate entry in this treatment section.

Standard Medical Treatments

Because anxiety symptoms may be caused by or related to other serious medical problems, it is essential to consult your physician about proper treatment. You may suffer an upset stomach or nausea when you are under stress, but the underlying cause of the symptoms may be an ulcer or a thyroid problem, conditions that require appropriate medication or other medical procedures. Even with conditions caused entirely by anxiety, such as panic disorder, your doctor may prescribe anti-anxiety drugs, such as benzodiazepine or buspirone; heterocyclic antidepressants; or selective serotonin reuptake inhibitors.[6]

But standard medical treatments are not the only answer. With most types of anxiety—regardless of whether or not the patient is being treated with standard methods, such as with a prescription drug—a mind body approach may serve as a significant player in the treatment plan.[7]

Scientific Proof for Mind Body Approaches

Our studies at the Benson-Henry Institute show that mind body interventions have a significant influence on at least two common symptoms of anxiety. First, with such mind body treatments, pounding heartbeats (palpitations) decline from a rate of once or twice a month to less than once a month. We have determined that there is less than a one-in-1,000 probability that these findings are due to chance. Our research also shows that shortness of breath decreased noticeably as a result of mind body treatments.[8]

The medical literature supporting our recent findings is extensive. My own collaborations with scientists over the years have often featured the use of mind body techniques to counter various types of anxiety. In an early study published in 1978 in *Psychotherapy and Psychosomatics,* I headed a team from the Harvard Medical School and Beth Israel Hospital in Boston that explored in 32 patients how two types of mind body techniques might be used to counter anxiety.[9]

The first technique involved a simple method of self-hypnosis; the second required an elicitation of the relaxation response using an approach similar to what we use in Phase One of our mind body treatment protocol. The patients were instructed to practice their assigned technique—self-hypnosis or evoking the relaxation response—daily for eight weeks. We found essentially no difference between the two techniques in therapeutic efficacy: Psychiatric assessments revealed an overall improvement in 34 percent of the patients, and a self-rating assessment indicated improvement in 63 percent. We concluded that "the meditational and self-hypnosis techniques employed in this investigation are simple to use and effective in the therapy of anxiety."

The implications for such findings also reach into the workplace. Working under Patricia Carrington of Princeton University, several other scientists and I explored how meditation-relaxation techniques might apply to the management of stress in organizational settings. Specifically, we focused on a stress-reduction program involving 154 New York Telephone employees.[10]

The participants, who consisted of 70 men and 84 women ranging in age from 22 to 65 years, were divided into three different mind body treatment groups and a control group. The three treatment groups were taught a progressive muscle relaxation technique, the standard relaxation response technique we use for Phase One of our Benson-Henry Protocol, or a different meditation technique devised by Carrington. After five and a half months, all the groups showed clinical improvement in self-reported symptoms of stress. We concluded, "The safe and inexpensive semi-automated meditation training has considerable value for stress-management programs in organization settings."

A related study, on which I collaborated with Ruanne K. Peters of the Harvard School of Public Health and which we described in the *Harvard Business Review*,[11] showed how corporate employees could lower their blood pressure and improve their general physical and psychological health through daily use of the relaxation response. The investigation compared a group who regularly took a "relaxation response break" with a second group that just sat quietly and with a third group that pursued normal daily activities. The group that elicited the relaxation response performed this exercise an average of 8.5 times per week for eight weeks.

After eight weeks, the relaxation response group had significantly lower blood pressure levels than the other two groups. They reported fewer headaches and backaches, less nausea and diarrhea, less insomnia, and fewer nervous habits that are associated with stress responses. The relaxation response group rated themselves as having increased their performance levels at work above the levels reported by those in the other two groups.[12]

Our later research and medical reports have confirmed that mind body techniques can be highly effective in reducing the impact of other types of environmental stress, including those listed on the classic Holmes-Rahe scale of stressful events, first published in 1967. This scale lists the top five stressful events in life as including death of a spouse, divorce, marital separation, serving a jail term, and death of a close family member.[13] In an article in *Behavioral and Biological Medicine,* I explored how mind body techniques can be used to treat anxiety symptoms stemming from these and other stressful events.

Possible Mind Body Treatments

As you know from the discussion in Chapter 6 (page 95), you have several options in applying an effective mind body treatment to help counter certain problems with anxiety. But they should all include Phase One and Phase Two of the Benson-Henry Protocol, which is summarized on page 111 of this chapter.

A simple illustration of how mind body techniques can lower anxiety involved a college student, Charles, who had considerable difficulty taking standardized tests, such as the GRE and the GMAT. Charles was a good student who earned well-above-average grades. During tutoring for these exams he displayed a firm grasp of the material, but when he took the standardized tests he consistently performed far below his potential.

Upon questioning, Charles said that he felt nervous before and during the tests—so nervous, in fact, that he "couldn't think straight." He said that even when he was taking an occasional practice test under timed conditions, he could feel his heart pounding and his breath coming in short bursts. With a mind body counselor, he began to take steps to counter his performance anxiety. The treatment program consisted of the following:

First, he went through a desensitization procedure, which involved taking many practice tests under timed conditions. He signed up to take as many standardized tests as he could. The rationale for this approach, which was consistent with common cognitive restructuring programs, was to make the test taking so routine that his nerves lost much of their sensitivity to the fear of undergoing an examination.

In addition, Charles was taught Phase One and Phase Two of our mind body protocol. In the 12-to-15-minute period of Phase One, he elicited the relaxation response by using the word *one*. In Phase Two, he took 8 to 10 minutes to visualize himself in school situations that he enjoyed, such as intramural sports, leisurely meals with friends, or intellectually stimulating discussions. He did *not* see himself in a test-taking situation; that mental picture would have been likely to raise his anxiety levels.

After eight days of engaging in our two-phase mind body protocol, Charles reported that he felt more relaxed during timed practice tests. "Now, I really don't feel any nerves at all," he reported.

This progress encouraged him to continue with his mind body exercises. Most important of all, when he took an actual GRE a few weeks later, his anxiety levels were much lower, and his score on the section of the test on which he had focused increased significantly.

But even though our mind body protocol works quite well for many types of anxiety, there is one anxiety-specific danger area—an "anxiety paradox"—that you should avoid if you want to achieve the maximum effect of the treatment.

The Anxiety Paradox

Ironically, when you are employing a mind body technique to counter anxiety, the anxiety may actually increase in some cases. This reverse effect of the treatment is especially common in the early stages of learning the two-phase approach.

A particular concern may arise with the use of certain focus words. Patients have reported that a word or phrase that would normally be associated with inner peace and calm, such as words out of the person's worship tradition, may have the opposite impact. One female editor, Randy, reported that saying silently, "God loves me," actually increased her anxiety levels and made it impossible to rid her mind of distracting thoughts.

Randy was instructed to experiment until she found a focus device that would carry no emotional weight, positive or negative. She eventually decided not to use a word or phrase for her focus, but instead just to concentrate on physical factors—relaxing her muscles, breathing regularly, and watching the specks moving behind her closed eyelids. This nonverbal approach helped calm her down and made it easier for her to turn away from distracting thoughts.

What exactly was happening in this case?

Most likely, Randy slipped into a subtle "performance anxiety" related to her belief system. By invoking the name of God in Phase One, she may have assumed that she had to perform up to God's standards with this exercise. Or she may have felt she was putting God "on the line," so to speak. As a result, she avoided references to her belief system in Phase One. Later, as she became more comfortable with the two-phase mind body protocol, she found it easier to return to a spiritually linked focus word or phase.

I sometimes say that it's necessary at the outset of the exercise for some patients to do a "prefrontal lobotomy" on their everyday thoughts—to cut them completely out of the mind—and that may include everyday religious thoughts. Anxiety is a rather devious condition that is particularly susceptible to religious beliefs. But as an individual becomes more accustomed to employing our two-phase treatment protocol, mind body performance anxiety tends to recede, and the door opens to the use of spiritual imagery and focus words.

So if you have chosen a spiritual focus word for Phase One but then find your anxiety levels increase, just put aside the spiritually oriented language and focus on your breathing and/or progressive muscle relaxation. If you're like most people, you may be able to return to the spiritual focus later, when you have become more used to the Benson-Henry Protocol.

Depression

Symptoms

More than 20 million Americans suffer from depression, according to the National Institutes of Health.[14] Symptoms may include a range of feelings and physical manifestations, including the following:

- frequent or constant feelings of sadness;
- lack of an appetite;
- insomnia or, conversely, a tendency to sleep unusually long hours or a consistent reluctance to get out of bed;
- a sense that life isn't really worth living;
- an unusual loss of weight (five or more pounds) without any attempt at a reduction program;
- a reduction in your activities or a regular feeling of being immobilized;
- a lack of a desire to socialize with others; and
- a lack of interest in sex.

Standard Medical Treatments

Mild depression, a condition that may last for months, is characterized by many of the symptoms listed above but does not result in a significant loss of the ability to function. Common treatments include the prescription of stimulants such as methylphenidate (Ritalin), especially for older people. The downside is that stimulants used in mild depression may cause mental confusion or emotional agitation.

Major depression involves the above symptoms but may also be characterized by inability to function in daily tasks, and sometimes by suicidal tendencies. A variety of antidepressant drugs may be used for treatment. These include the selective serotonin reuptake inhibitors (SSRI), such as fluoxetine and sertraline, and the heterocyclic antidepressants (HCA), such as trazodone, imipramine, and amitriptyline. Another class of strong drugs that may be prescribed are the monoamine oxidase inhibitors (MAOI).

But side effects for these medications for major depression can be substantial. Depending on the drug, they include disruption of sleep, reduced sexual response, dizziness, slowing of urination in men with enlarged prostates, dry mouth, and a sense of grogginess that accompanies being overly sedated. Stronger drugs also open the door to serious drug interactions. The MAOI class of medications may be associated with high blood pressure in those taking buspirone, seizures and comas in those taking meperidine, or altered consciousness in those taking tricyclic or heterocyclic antidepressants.

In addition, patients who stop taking antidepressant drugs are prone to withdrawal symptoms such as headaches, nausea, and dizziness. These patients may also experience mental difficulties such as confusion, memory loss, or nightmares.

Some depressed patients may be referred to electroconvulsive therapy (ECT), or shock treatments. In this type of therapy, the patient is anesthetized, electrodes are placed on the head, and electrical currents are sent through the scalp, causing a brief seizure. Side effects include short-term memory loss, sore muscles, and headaches.

Fortunately, for many cases of depression a more benign, mind body treatment may be appropriate—an alternative that may enable you to reduce your antidepressant medication.

Scientific Proof for Mind Body Approaches

Researchers recognize that depression can be relieved in up to 50 percent of patients by the expectation and belief that are associated with the placebo effect, and not just by drugs.[15] When drugs are used, researchers have determined that the positive response of patients to antidepressant medications may be due to the expectation-belief features of the placebo response rather than to the drug itself.[16] Perhaps most important for the average patient, the impact of the placebo on depression can have a relatively long-lasting effect—but usually without side effects of medications.[17]

What is the physiologic explanation for the power of the expectation-belief factor?

Researchers have done studies comparing the placebo effect to the effects of a wide variety of antidepressant drugs, including the selective serotonin reuptake inhibitors, such as sertraline and fluoxetine. These studies have consistently revealed the power of the placebo effect in relieving depression. Patients report that the antidepressant drugs are slightly more effective than the placebos, but patients generally tolerate the placebos better than the drugs.

PET scans (positron-emission tomography) involve a sectional, computerized scan of the body using radioisotopes injected into the bloodstream. When this equipment has been used to study the human brain, the results shown in the brain after taking a placebo are consistent with changes after taking real drugs. Furthermore, brain scans have shown significant activity in those parts of the brain involved in the release of morphine-like opioid neurotransmitters, such as endorphins, which can relieve or eliminate pain. In addition, scientists have discovered that in combating depression, placebos stimulate the natural release of the neurotransmitter serotonin.[18]

Making "real-time" computerized images of the functioning brain in depressed patients has shown that specific changes occur in the brain when expectation and belief are in operation.[19] The research also suggests that a wide variety of practical treatment techniques can work to trigger positive belief and expectation in alleviating depression.

A 2007 study published in *Behaviour Research and Therapy,* which evaluated the impact of several treatment interventions to treat depression in adolescents, illustrates this point. The interventions included writing, reading, cognitive behavior therapy, and supportive group intervention.[20] The research showed that the controls received no benefits, while *all of the active interventions* worked to significantly reduce depressive symptoms by the end of the study. The authors concluded that a major component in the success of these interventions may have been the *expectation* on the part of participants that their intervention would work.

Possible Mind Body Treatments

You should begin your mind body treatment with the two-phase Benson-Henry Protocol summarized on page 111.

In Phase One, which will require about 12 to 15 minutes, you change your physiology and alter your gene activity—or "turn on" healthy gene activity and "turn off" unhealthy activity—by evoking the relaxation response. As the relaxation response takes hold of your entire body and your brain becomes calmer, a mind-opening effect occurs, leaving you in a state where you are better prepared to focus fully on healthy thoughts and memories. Relief from your symptoms of depression should begin during this first phase.

With your mind calmer and more open, you are ready to begin Phase Two of the mind body healing process for treating depression. During the 8 to 10 minutes of Phase Two visualization, see yourself in a state of health without the symptoms of depression. We encourage you to think back on a specific time when you remember that you were quite happy or joyous. In effect you "remember wellness"—a period when you were healthy, upbeat, and satisfied with your life and relationships. On the whole, you recall that you were much more "up" than "down" emotionally.

If possible, link your visualization to your personal philosophy of life, as a way to bolster your state of positive expectation and belief. Suppose, for instance, that you have become firmly convinced that a positive, "can-do" attitude toward life will be more likely to result in your personal happiness and success than a more morose or negative outlook—even if the upbeat approach may sometimes seem unrealistic or Pollyannaish. To counter depression using this worldview, you might draw a mental picture of yourself in a joyous movie scene, such as one of those depicted in the musical *The Sound of Music*. While this suggestion may seem silly to some, you should be motivated by the visualization approach that will *work for you*—not some less effective approach that you think might merit the approval of others. Remember: Your objective is to be healed of your depression, not to secure the approval of anyone else.

Finally, always bring your physician into the mind body healing process. Any alleviation of the symptoms could cause your physician to consider prescribing lower doses of any antidepressant drug you are taking, or eliminating the drug entirely.

Hypertension (High Blood Pressure)

Symptoms

Hypertension, or high blood pressure, which affects more than 60 million Americans according to various estimates, has no symptoms until
it reaches dangerously high or destructive levels. The condition has
rightly been labeled a "silent killer." In extreme cases, such symptoms as
severe headache, dizziness, eyestrain, nosebleed, or fatigue may occur.
But the overwhelming majority of those with hypertension have no
symptoms.

The only way to determine whether your blood pressure is high is
to have it measured with a sphygmomanometer (arm-cuff apparatus)
or another computerized medical device. Current recommendations
are that blood pressure should ideally be lower than 120/80 mm Hg
(the upper or first figure is known as the systolic pressure while the
lower figure is the diastolic pressure).

Systolic pressure from 120 to 139 and/or diastolic pressure from
80 to 89 are considered "prehypertensive" and pose an increased risk
of more severe hypertension. Systolic pressure from 140 to 159 and/or
diastolic pressure from 90 to 99 are classified as "Stage 1 hypertension,"
a level that will require medications if appropriate changes in lifestyle,
such as loss of weight or aerobic exercise, don't work. Readings of 160
systolic and/or 100 diastolic are classified as "Stage 2 hypertension"
and require drugs plus lifestyle changes.

If left untreated, hypertension may lead to serious health problems, including stroke, heart attacks, and kidney failure.

Standard Medical Treatments

According to standard medical practice, physicians may prescribe a
wide variety of medications and lifestyle changes. For "prehypertension," physicians typically prescribe such lifestyle changes as weight loss;
aerobic or endurance exercise; avoidance of salt; reduction of excessive
alcohol intake; cessation of smoking; and relaxation exercises, including
the evocation of the relaxation response. Those patients with Stage 1 or

Stage 2 hypertension may be directed to take one or more antihypertensive drugs. These drugs include diuretics, ACE (angiotensin converting enzyme) inhibitors, beta-blockers, angiotensin-II receptor antagonists, calcium antagonists, and potassium-sparing agents.

Unfortunately, drugs tend to carry side effects. Depending on the antihypertensive medication, these effects might include dizziness (from hypotension, or too-low blood pressure), headache, fatigue, chest discomfort, persistent cough, sexual dysfunction, diarrhea, excessively fast heart rate (tachycardia), glucose intolerance, ankle swelling, and constipation.

Scientific Proof for Mind Body Approaches

A recently described effect of both strong expectation-belief and the relaxation response is that they trigger a release of nitric oxide in the body's cells, which serves as a vasodilator, an agent that expands the blood vessels.[21] This dilation process can be highly effective in reducing blood pressure. In fact, many of the most effective new antihypertensive drugs, such as ACE inhibitors, are vasodilators. But any patient might ask quite reasonably, "Why not use a mind body approach—which operates as a vasodilator but has no side effects—rather than a vasodilator drug, which *does* have side effects?"

My published studies on this work—and parallel studies by other scientists—have spanned more than three decades, from 1974 to the present.[22] Because much hypertension can be traced to chronic stress, our Phase One and Two protocol, which can control stress, places at our disposal a powerful, if little used, medical tool to treat this pervasive disease.

So the scientific evidence clearly shows that 1) eliciting the relaxation response, 2) triggering the placebo effect, or 3) using both of these mind body approaches can lower blood pressure significantly.

Possible Mind Body Treatments

Your mind body treatment for hypertension should begin with the standard Benson-Henry Protocol summarized on page 111.

With hypertension, extensive research indicates that you should definitely employ Phase One of our basic mind body treatment protocol. Calm and open your mind and body by evoking the relaxation response, with all the genetic, molecular, and other beneficial physiologic changes that this process entails.

Phase Two, which involves visualization of an image based on past memory of good health, may not even be necessary: Many of our studies have shown that simply experiencing the relaxation response is often enough to lower blood pressure significantly.

On the other hand, the visualization phase can be quite powerful to the extent that it brings the placebo effect—or remembered wellness—into play. In most cases we would recommend that you employ Phase Two with hypertension, even if Phase One proves to be highly effective.

Specifically, after you have opened your mind to the relaxation response for about 15 minutes, spend about 10 more minutes picturing a pleasant, calm scene. Imagine yourself on a beach, with gentle waves washing over you. Or lie in a meadow in the mountains, with the trees moving softly overhead and birds singing in the background. Or you could imagine yourself just resting in the presence of God.

The important thing is that you choose a mental scene that is calm and stress free and, if possible, that conforms to your deepest personal beliefs. If you have a deep commitment to classical music, for instance, you might see—and mentally "hear"—yourself transported on notes from a piece by Mozart or Bach. This two-phase mind body protocol will place you in an ideal position to increase your body's output of nitric oxide, expand your blood vessels (vasodilation), and lower your blood pressure accordingly.

Consider the experience of one of my patients, whom I'll call Joan:

Joan, 68 years old, developed high blood pressure over a 10-year period—a Stage 2 condition of 164/80 mm Hg. She began taking two medications to control her hypertension, a calcium channel-blocker and an ACE (angiotensin converting enzyme) inhibitor. On these medications, her blood pressure decreased to 146/78, which was still in the hypertensive range. (You will recall that Stage 1 hypertension ranges from 140/90 to 159/99.) But she also suffered from drug side effects, including headaches, dizziness, excessive fatigue, and regular coughing spells.

We placed her on a relaxation response program, which involved eight weeks of eliciting the relaxation response once daily while listening to what we have called the "Olivia CD," a calming listening experience with soothing voices and sounds.* The disk both helped her elicit the relaxation response and encouraged her to visualize calming scenes, which reinforced the impact of the relaxation response.

As a result of this program, her blood pressure was lowered to 129/74. After continuing her mind body program over the next 8 to 12 weeks, she was able to maintain this lower level of blood pressure—and was able to discontinue her medications with no increase in blood pressure. The drug side effects also disappeared.

Joan became a case study in how the effective mind body treatment of hypertension can result in the complete elimination of anti-hypertensive drugs. The relaxation response—combined with the placebo effect—was as effective in treating high blood pressure as the two drugs she had been taking.

Joan's experience is significant for another reason. Her condition, isolated systolic hypertension—or elevation of the "upper" or "first" number in the blood pressure measurement—is a prevalent condition in people over age 65. More than 10 million Americans suffer from this form of hypertension. Scientific research has proven that there is no effective drug therapy for this problem, even though drugs with serious side effects continue to be prescribed and used for this age group. In contrast, our research published in 2008 has shown that our mind body management approach lowers the systolic pressure on average by 10 mm Hg.[23] Furthermore, we found that those practicing mind body treatments may often be able to decrease or even eliminate hypertensive medication.

---

* See the description of the Olivia CD in Chapter 2, page 24.

Infertility (Stress-Related)

Symptoms

Infertility refers to the inability to conceive and bear children. About one-third of infertility cases arise from problems on the male side, such as the inability to produce enough sperm. Another third of these problems can be traced to the female, including blockages or other difficulties with the fallopian tubes, the channels through which the eggs move to the womb, the "meeting place" for the egg and sperm.[24] The remaining third of infertility situations are often a mystery, though a significant portion of these "unknown" cases may be stress-related. The stress may come from either the female or the male, or from the dynamic involving their relationship.

Standard Medical Treatments

A variety of fertility treatments have arisen in recent years for both men and women. Women may be prescribed fertility drugs such as follicle-stimulating hormone, luteinizing hormone, bromocriptine, and clomiphene citrate. In various ways, these drugs cause the ovaries to release eggs. Unfortunately, these drugs may carry significant side effects. Depending on the drug, these side effects may include hot flashes, nausea, dizziness, or various pains.

In men, treatments may include antibiotics for prostate or other infections that can cause infertility, or surgery to correct such problems as varicoceles, varicose veins in the testicles that cause swelling and may impede sperm movement.

If these medical interventions do not work, another possibility involves what is called "assisted reproductive technology," including in vitro fertilization and other methods that feature manipulation of the sperm and eggs so as to induce pregnancy.[25] With in vitro fertilization, sperm and eggs are harvested from the couple and placed into a dish, where fertilization takes place. Then the healthiest fertilized eggs are placed into the woman's uterus (womb) through a catheter, and progesterone is administered to the woman to encourage implantation of the embryo. If the procedure is successful, a normal pregnancy begins.

In addition to these drug and surgical approaches, the third option may involve lifestyle adjustments, including weight loss, stopping smoking, eliminating alcohol usage, and better stress management, according to advice given in the *Harvard Medical School Family Health Guide* by infertility expert Alice Domar of the Beth Israel Deaconess Medical Center, the Harvard Medical School, and our Institute.[26]

Scientific Proof for Mind Body Approaches

We introduced research on page 69 showing that stress reduction is associated with increased fertility, in particular a 1990 investigation, conducted by Domar, in which we found that 34 percent of 54 previously infertile women became pregnant after going through a 10-week program in which they learned to elicit the relaxation response.[27]

Confirming these conclusions in 1992 in *Fertility and Sterility,* our team found that another group of 52 infertile women experienced statistically significant decreases in anxiety, depression, confusion, bewilderment, and anger after a relaxation response program. In this investigation, 32 percent of the women became pregnant within six months of completing the program.[28]

Other studies, going back at least to 1993, have supported the findings that stress-reduction programs—especially those involving the relaxation response—can be quite helpful in overcoming infertility.[29]

Possible Mind Body Treatments

Begin with our two-phase Benson-Henry Protocol summarized on page 111.

If you are confronting infertility, continue with any medical interventions directed by your physician. But in addition, a mind body approach is advisable to lower stress levels and increase the potential for a pregnancy. In light of our research in this area, a combination treatment, including both ordinary medical approaches and the relaxation response, may very well increase your chances to have a child.

In Phase Two, your visualizations may include any comforting or calming imagery—but should *not* focus on your failure to conceive. Don't picture yourself as being infertile and then becoming pregnant and having a child. Such an approach would be more likely to increase rather than reduce your stress levels. Instead, you might recall a particularly happy and peaceful experience you have had recently that is unrelated to your particular medical problem.

One infertility patient, for instance, remembered how peaceful it often was for her to go away on a business retreat, sink down on a bed in her hotel room, and forget the cares of work, home, and family. The ostensible purpose of such trips for her and her colleagues was to brainstorm about solutions to problems at work, an activity that may sound a lot like high-pressure work. But in fact, these away-from-the-home-office conferences relaxed her better than any vacation.

"On a regular vacation, I tend to get more stressed out than I do when I'm just staying home—because I'm always worrying about the work I've left behind," she said. "So remembering one of those experiences would probably work against any feelings of inner calm or peace."

In contrast, bringing up mental images of one of the recent business retreats increased her level of emotional calm immeasurably. This kind of visualization, unattached to any particular worry about pregnancy, may foster an overall calming and sense of relaxation—and help with stress-related fertility problems.

Insomnia

Symptoms

Insomnia refers to the inability to get to sleep in a reasonable amount of time or an inability to get a good night's rest because of interrupted sleep.[30] A common principle is that if it takes you 30 minutes or longer to get to sleep on a regular basis, you have insomnia. In contrast, you do not have insomnia if you usually get to sleep in 20 minutes or less.

Related symptoms or signs of insomnia include daytime drowsiness, diminished productivity, and increased absenteeism at work.

Although most adults sleep seven to eight hours per night, the healthiest sleep patterns appear to range from about five to nine hours per night.[31] A 2006 Columbia University study published in *Hypertension* revealed that those who sleep five hours or less per night are at higher risk for hypertension.[32] Those who sleep less than five or more than nine hours per night may be at risk for shorter lives.

Researchers at our Institute have suggested that about 20 to 40 percent of adults have trouble sleeping, and one in six regards insomnia as a serious problem. In fact, some experts believe that insomnia is the second most prevalent health complaint after pain.[33]

Standard Medical Treatments

Medical caregivers use a variety of approaches to combat insomnia but with varying degrees of success. Prescription drugs such as the benzodiazepines may help for a short time, but then they tend to become less effective. Drugs such as the heterocyclic antidepressants may also be prescribed, but they may cause side effects, such as constipation, weight gain, dizziness, or even a decreased ability to sleep.

Because drug therapy typically does not work for most patients on a long-term basis and also carries many side effects, physicians often rely on lifestyle changes, such as conditioning the patient to use the bed only for sleep or sex (see the description of lifestyle and mind body treatments below). Many experts say that the most effective long-term approach for most people may involve lifestyle adaptations plus mind body techniques, including the evocation of the relaxation response.[34]

Scientific Proof for Mind Body Approaches

In a 2009 study led by Marlene Samuelson and Megan Foret at the Benson-Henry Institute, we determined that insomnia was one of the conditions that proved most responsive to mind body interventions.[35] Specifically, we found that as a result of 12 weeks of mind body treatments, frequency of insomnia declined from nearly twice a week to about once a week: the occurrence rate was almost cut in half. Our investigation also showed that the likelihood was less than one in 1,000 that these improvements were due to chance.

A number of earlier studies, which we have explained in Chapter 4, pages 57–70, support these recent findings. At the risk of being redundant, we have summarized some of that material below to help reinforce our point that there is indeed strong scientific support for the mind body approach to insomnia.

In a study published in 1993, a team at our Institute led by Gregg Jacobs explored ways to reduce the time it takes for an individual to move from being fully awake to entering the first stages of sleep.[36] As indicated above, the usual rule is that an insomniac takes 30 minutes or longer to get to sleep, while the go-to-sleep time for noncomplaining sleepers is 20 minutes or less.

In this study, participants were divided into two groups. One group was assigned to a program that involved lifestyle adjustments and lessons in "sleep hygiene" techniques, such as:

- avoiding evening use of alcohol, nicotine, and caffeine;
- increasing daily exercise but not too close to bedtime (a general rule of thumb is that vigorous exercise should be avoided within three hours of bedtime);
- establishing a regular routine just before bedtime, such as going to bed at the same time every night;
- using the bed and bedroom only for sleep and sex;
- arising at the same time every morning;
- going to bed only when sleepy;
- avoiding daytime naps; and
- using pleasant background noise to mask any sleep-disruptive noises.

The other group of participants was taught these stimulus control techniques plus the evocation of the relaxation response. All subjects underwent a 10-week period of training, and also a post-treatment follow-up for one month.

Both groups improved significantly in reducing the amount of time they took to get to sleep, but the group that had used the relaxation response did better. On average, they experienced a decline in sleep-onset time from more than 77 minutes to 17.5 minutes during the post-test period.

In another insomnia study conducted in 1996, Jacobs, Richard Friedman, and I found that an approach to insomnia that used lifestyle changes, the relaxation response, and various other cognitive restructuring techniques enabled over 90 percent of the participants who were using sleep medications to either eliminate or reduce their drug use.[37]

Possible Mind Body Treatments

To treat your insomnia, begin practicing the two-phase Benson-Henry Protocol summarized on page 111.

In light of the research and clinical experience in this area, we also recommend the following approach to treating your insomnia:

The Role of Posture

Because posture is a primary consideration when you want to fall asleep, you will need to alter our usual instructions about the two-phase mind body treatment protocol. Normally, we recommend that in Phase One you assume a comfortable *sitting* position. One of the reasons is to be sure you stay awake! Sitting in a chair, standing and swaying, sitting cross-legged on the floor, and kneeling are meditational or prayerful postures that have evolved over millennia, in part to keep practitioners from falling asleep.

But in treating insomnia, your objective is different: You want to assume a posture that will help you fall asleep, and that means it is necessary for you to *lie down* as you use the standard relaxation response instructions. As you break the train of everyday thought in a reclining posture, the stimuli traveling from your mind to your body will typically trigger physiologic responses and brain waves that produce sleep instead of a wakeful calmness.

A peculiar problem that often occurs as you're trying to drift off to sleep is that you may lapse into a foggy state, not quite awake or asleep, during which anxious thoughts—such as "I'm still not asleep and I have to get up in two hours!"—arouse you and keep you awake. In this foggy state, you may also find it particularly hard to center on your focus word or phrase.

As an antidote, most patients find that all they have to do is condition themselves with regular practice of the two-phase mind body exercise during their wakeful hours. With that training, they are much more likely to be able to turn away from distractions with an "Oh well"; break the train of everyday thought; and, because of the reclining position, fall asleep.

For the Phase Two visualization, you have a range of possibilities when dealing with insomnia. You might picture yourself floating on a cloud, completely relaxed—and hold that image for the recommended 8 to 10 minutes. Or you might imagine yourself floating in a warm pool of water. Or you might recall a sleep-enhancing experience you have had in a natural setting; perhaps you lay down under a tree or on a seashore to rest, and your eyes grew so heavy that you had no choice but to fall asleep. This "remembered wellness" thought could carry sufficient suggestive power to cause you to become drowsy.

Another possibility is the classic "sheep-counting" method, which fits nicely into our two-phase paradigm. Try some repetitive counting in your mind, starting with the number one and going forward, or starting with 100 and counting backward. When you do this, do not feel that you have to hurry or get all the numbers exactly in order. If a distracting thought enters your mind and you lose your place in the counting sequence, don't become concerned. Simply think, "Oh well," pick any number, and start your count from that point.

In addition to using our basic two-phase mind body protocol to treat insomnia, you should find it helpful to employ some of the lifestyle adjustments mentioned in our research studies summarized above and also in Chapter 4, page 64.[38] You will recall that these adjustments include such steps as avoiding stimulants and exercise just before bedtime, establishing a regular pre-sleep routine, and using the bedroom and bed only for sleep and sex. You might use the list of these lifestyle changes as a personal checklist—in combination with the basic two-phase protocol—to enhance your own ability to achieve better sleep.

Menopausal, Perimenopausal, and Breast Cancer Hot Flashes

Symptoms

Menopause, which is often defined as a lack of menstrual periods for one straight year, may begin for women in their mid-40s. Menopause tends to end around age 50, though the age range varies widely, depending on the individual.[39] This "change of life" in older women is caused by a decline in estrogen output, which marks the end of the reproductive or childbearing years.

Symptoms may include irregular periods, "hot flashes" (a sense of marked changes in body temperature), insomnia, excessive perspiration ("night sweats") at night, dryness of the vagina, changes in body-fat distribution, varying degrees of incontinence, sexual dysfunction, and mood swings.

Standard Medical Treatments

In treating menopausal hot flashes and related symptoms, physicians may prescribe hormone replacement therapy, including the administration of estrogen and progesterone. However, in recent years, doctors have been less likely to advocate this treatment because of the possibility of serious side effects, such as an increased risk of breast cancer, strokes, blood clots, or gallbladder problems. Also, your physician may recommend special exercises, such as Kegel exercises for pelvic strengthening to help control incontinence, estrogen ointments for vaginal dryness, and dressing in clothing layers to enable you to better control the effect of hot flashes.[40]

In addition to these approaches, a growing body of scientific evidence shows that mind body techniques may be quite effective in controlling such menopausal symptoms as hot flashes.

Scientific Proof for Mind Body Approaches

Research from our Institute has revealed some promising findings with regard to the application of mind body approaches to control menopausal symptoms.[41] In a 1996 report in the *Journal of Psychosomatic Obstetrics and Gynecology,* a team led by J. H. Irvin and A. D. Domar studied a group of 33 women, ranging in age from 44 to 66 years, who had gone a minimum of six months without a menstrual period.[42] Also, the women had all experienced at least five hot flashes during a 24-hour period and were not using hormone replacement therapy.

For the 10-week study, the women were randomly assigned to one of three groups: a relaxation response training group, a reading group, and a control group. The researchers found that the relaxation response group, in comparison with the other groups, showed "significant reductions in hot flash intensity . . . tension-anxiety . . . and depression."

Many other investigations have supported our findings:

- A 2006 study at the University of Massachusetts Medical School of 15 female volunteers focused on a possible link between hot flashes and stress, especially stress in women with lower coping abilities. The volunteers reported a minimum of seven moderate-to-severe hot flashes per day at the beginning of the study. Then the participants were assigned to eight weekly classes teaching a stress-reduction technique.

  The researchers found that the women's scores on quality-of-life measures increased significantly, and their median hot-flash severity decreased by 40 percent over the course of the 11-week assessment period. The authors concluded that the results "provide preliminary positive evidence of the feasibility and efficacy of MBSR [a mindfulness-based stress-reduction program] in supporting women who are experiencing severe HFs [hot flashes]...."[43]

- A 2008 report in the *Journal of Managed Care Pharmacy* noted that vasomotor symptoms, such as hot flashes and "night sweats," are the most bothersome symptoms of menopause, affecting an estimated 75 percent of women over 50 years of age.[44]

    The authors recommended making lifestyle changes—such as following relaxation techniques—to help reduce the risk of hot flashes and night sweats. They also said that these vasomotor symptoms may be alleviated by other lifestyle adjustments, such as regular physical activity, weight loss, and smoking cessation. They recommended that hormone replacement therapy be used at the lowest effective dose for the shortest period possible, to avoid the risk of side effects.

The Perimenopausal and Breast Cancer Issues

Hot flashes may also occur among women in the premenopause (perimenopausal) stage of life and among those who have had breast cancer. Perimenopause has been defined as the time frame before a woman's periods cease but after they start to become irregular.[45] Hot flashes are experienced by an estimated 52 percent of perimenopausal women and about 70 percent of those who have had breast cancer.[46]

In a 2008 British study, researchers conducted a randomized controlled trial of 150 women with breast cancer who experienced hot flashes. The intervention (treatment) group was given one relaxation training session and was instructed to use relaxation practice tapes daily at home for one month. The control group received no such instruction. The researchers found that the incidence, severity, and distress caused by hot flashes declined significantly over a one-month period in the relaxation group, in comparison with the control group. The researchers concluded "relaxation may be a useful component of a program of measures to relieve hot flashes in women with primary breast cancer."[47]

A 2008 review in *Menopause* reported on bothersome hot flashes in menopausal women and also in breast cancer survivors. The article focused on 14 studies involving 475 patients. Noting that most drug interventions and herbal therapies for hot flashes are limited because of side effects or ineffectiveness, the authors concluded, "psycho-educational interventions, including relaxation, seem to alleviate hot flashes in menopausal women and breast cancer survivors. . . ."[48]

Such results suggest that the two-phase mind body protocol that we recommend in this book—a protocol that features the elicitation of the relaxation response in Phase One and appropriate visualization in Phase Two—could be quite useful for women with menopausal, perimenopausal, and breast cancer hot flashes and with related symptoms, such as night sweats.

Possible Mind Body Treatments

To treat hot flashes and related symptoms, practice daily the two-phase Benson-Henry Protocol summarized on page 111.

As you practice Phase Two visualization, you might combine the Phase One relaxation response with visualization using this approach:

Proceed through the muscle relaxation procedure in Phase One. Then, as you focus on your breathing, choose a "low-temperature" focus word like *cool* or *breeze.* As you repeat the word, allow your mind to wander over mental pictures or other associations that reaffirm your focus. You will note that elsewhere in this book, we have suggested that your focus words should not only conform to your belief system but should also be neutral. In this case, however, the choice of a focus word suggesting the health state you want may be preferable.

For example, you might find yourself remembering a cool, dry lounge you recall from a vacation hotel you visited. Or you might also imagine a particularly refreshing drink as you are sitting there in the lounge. Linger a few moments in that scene, just enjoying the pleasant, breezy atmosphere.

Or your imagination may transport you to a windy mountaintop or winter scene, which you remember as particularly invigorating and inspiring. If you find that the "remembered wellness" image that has come to mind is particularly enjoyable or pleasurable, don't be in a hurry to leave it. Stay there for a while in your mind's eye, and examine the particulars of the terrain or scenery.

If at any point you find your mind drifting away from the pleasant scene onto more mundane matters of life, return to your focus word and concentrate on your breathing. As with other uses of our two-phase protocol, if distracting thoughts keep intruding, just say, "Oh well," and return to your focus word. Hold those focus words and "cool" images and memories in your mind for the full 20 to 25 minutes of the mind body protocol.

You will note that in this case we have combined Phases One and Two, allowing elements of each to overlap. Exercising such flexibility in your protocol will become easier the more experienced you become in using your mind body techniques. Of course, if you prefer to keep the two phases separate, that's quite acceptable as well. You could spend 12 to 15 minutes with your focus word, such as *cool* or *breeze,* and then finish with 8 to 10 minutes of a visualization session, which might involve a cool, refreshing scene or memory. Your total treatment time would be the same as that for the more flexible approach we have just suggested for hot flashes: 20 to 25 minutes.

There is no one "correct" way to take advantage of the two-phase protocol for hot flashes—or for any other medical condition, for that matter. As you seek the best mind body treatment for yourself, just be sure that you achieve the three basic objectives mentioned in our protocol summaries: 1) break the pattern of everyday thoughts and concerns; 2) maintain a passive, "oh well" attitude toward distracting thoughts; and 3) devote sufficient time to each session—a total of about 20 to 25 minutes for the entire protocol.

Nausea

Symptoms

Nausea, the urge to vomit, may occur for a wide variety of reasons. Serious causes, which require medical evaluation and treatment, include such conditions as nausea following a head injury; nausea accompanied by other symptoms, such as blood in the vomit or stool; or nausea that persists for several days.[49]

Nausea may also occur during stressful situations, such as those involving a need to make a public presentation or to deal with another high-pressure professional or personal situation. Examples include a dreaded interview with the boss or a confrontation with a family member. Nausea may also be caused by an intensely unpleasant odor or sight, or the anticipation of some distasteful event or responsibility, such as receiving chemotherapy.[50]

Standard Medical Treatments

Medical treatment will be required if the nausea follows head trauma or other injury. But nausea that arises primarily from stress or from anticipating a stressful situation can often be treated by the mind body approaches we advocate in this book.

Scientific Proof for Mind Body Approaches

Our studies at the Benson-Henry Institute have shown that nausea is one of the medical conditions that responds best to mind body therapy. In our 2009 study led by Marlene Samuelson and Megan Foret of the Benson-Henry Institute, we found that nausea symptoms decreased dramatically in frequency after patients learned to elicit the relaxation response. The participants, who were trained over 12 weeks in twice-weekly two-and-a-half-hour sessions, reduced their average occurrence of nausea from once or twice a month to less than once a month. We also found that the probability that this improvement had occurred by chance was less than one in 1,000.[51]

In addition to general, stress-related causes of nausea, a body of research shows that mind body therapy, including relaxation training, can help cancer patients on chemotherapy to manage their feelings of nausea.

- A 2007 study published in the *Journal of the National Comprehensive Cancer Network* concluded that behavioral interventions—"especially progressive muscle relaxation training and systematic desensitization"*—should be considered important methods for preventing and treating anticipatory nausea (nausea that arises in anticipation of chemotherapy that hasn't yet been administered) and vomiting by chemotherapy patients.[52]
- A 2005 South Korean study assessed the effectiveness of training in progressive muscle relaxation and guided imagery as treatments for nausea and vomiting before and after chemotherapy treatments for breast cancer.[53]

   The researchers found that both the progressive muscle relaxation and guided imagery groups were significantly less anxious, depressed, and hostile than the control group. They also found that patients using progressive muscle relaxation or guided imagery experienced significantly less anticipatory nausea and vomiting and also less post-procedure nausea and vomiting. Furthermore, the scientists determined through psychological measurements that six months after receiving the chemotherapy, the quality of life of the two experimental groups was higher than that of the control group.
- A joint study of 71 breast cancer patients, which involved an oncology unit at a university hospital in Hong Kong and researchers from the University of Nottingham in Great Britain, examined the effectiveness of progressive muscle relaxation training in managing nausea and vomiting during the use of chemotherapy.[54] In

---

* Progressive muscular relaxation training evokes the relaxation response and is one of the techniques we suggest for Phase One of our protocol.

this study, mind body techniques were employed in conjunction with anti-vomiting medications.

The investigators randomly assigned 38 of the participants to an experimental group who would employ mind body approaches, and placed the remaining 33 participants in a control group. The experimental group was provided training that was similar to what we recommend for our Phase One and Two protocols:

This group practiced progressive muscle relaxation techniques for one hour before chemotherapy and then daily for another five days, for a total of six progressive muscle relaxation training sessions. Each of the five sessions lasted for 25 minutes and was followed by five minutes of imagery techniques.

The researchers found that the progressive muscle relaxation training "considerably decreased" the duration of nausea and vomiting in the experimental group, as compared with the control group. Also, they noted that there were trends toward a lower frequency of nausea and vomiting. The investigators concluded that progressive muscle relaxation training is a useful technique to complement anti-vomiting drugs (antiemetics) for chemotherapy-induced nausea.

There is significant scientific support, then, for the use of mind body techniques for various types of nausea. Here are some suggestions about how to incorporate these techniques in your personal health plan.

Possible Mind Body Treatments

To treat nausea, begin to practice our two-phase Benson-Henry Protocol, which is summarized on page 111.

For a variety of reasons—including excessive stress or chemotherapy—you may find yourself feeling nauseated or sick to your stomach. In such a situation, try this self-treatment:

At the very first sign of nausea, or even the first worry about the *possibility* of nausea ("anticipatory nausea"), go to Phase One and evoke the relaxation response. After completing your 12- to 15-minute Phase One session, move to Phase Two mental imagery that features these two characteristics:

First, visualize yourself in a calm, peaceful environment that has nothing to do with the circumstances that have triggered, or threatened to trigger, your nausea. If you are about to undergo chemotherapy, picture yourself in a nonmedical, nonhospital environment. Or if you have an upset stomach because of some performance-related obligation you are confronting, in your mind's eye take yourself completely away from the stressful situation.

Second, as you picture yourself in this neutral setting, see yourself breathing easily and regularly. Then do a reality check: Be sure that you *really are* breathing this way. Nausea and subsequent vomiting are usually associated with interruptions in regular breathing. If you can just maintain your normal breathing rhythm, you will be more likely to reduce or eliminate your feelings of nausea.

Pain—General

Symptoms

One of nature's most important mechanisms that signal danger to human health, pain can cause us to avoid imminent danger (such as a scorching fire) or to seek immediate medical attention. Nerve endings or pain "fibers" transmit a sensation up the brain, causing us to wince, cry, or scream, depending on the intensity of the stimulus. But pain involves much more than simple physiologic reactions.

Pain has been defined by the International Association for the Study of Pain as an "unpleasant sensory and emotional experience associated with actual or potential tissue damage, or described in terms of such damage. . . . Pain is always subjective. Each individual learns the application of the word through experiences related to injury in early life. . . . It is unquestionably a sensation in a part or parts of the body, but it is also always unpleasant and therefore also an emotional experience."[55]

A more precise definition is difficult because, as indicated above, *pain is always subjective*. Physicians and medical researchers recognize this fact by evaluating the intensity or level of pain with subjective techniques, such as a "one-to-10" self-measurement or self-report scale, with which they ask patients to rate their pain as a "one" if it is insignificant or a "10" if it is unbearable. With such tools, pain researchers—and practicing physicians—are better able to determine how well drugs they are using may be alleviating certain pains.[56]

When you undergo a procedure at the dentist's office, for instance, the dentist or dental technician may ask whether you are experiencing pain in an effort to determine whether you need some local anesthetic. If you rate your pain at a "three" or "four," you will probably get through the procedure without a numbing agent. On the other hand, another patient may go through the same procedure and have substantially the same nerve physiology as yours but may rank the pain at a "seven" or "eight," a level that will probably require a painkilling medication. The procedures and the physical makeup are quite similar, but the *subjective perception* of the level of pain may be different in each person—and may require a different medical response.

Your symptoms may include pain of varying degrees in any part of the body, including the head, face, back, arms, abdomen, neck, shoulders, and legs. The pain may be classified as *chronic,* meaning that it has continued for six months or longer and tends not to respond well to standard medical treatments.[57] Usually chronic pain will begin with some physical stimulation, such as an athletic injury to the back or arthritis in a joint. Chronic pains may respond well to mind body treatments. Chronic pain will usually intensify if the patient is gripped by anxiety, fear, or a sense of helplessness.

Pain may also be classified as *acute,* or relatively short-term. Acute pain may result from a particular trauma or injury, such as a broken arm or a gunshot wound. Acute pains will typically be treated immediately with standard medical methods, such as prescription painkillers or surgery. But mind body approaches—including our two-phase protocol—can often be quite helpful in alleviating the intensity of the short-term pain and in easing or preventing the onset of chronic pain from the injury.

Standard Medical Treatments

The usual treatment for chronic pain—and for many serious acute pains—is prescription or over-the-counter painkillers or analgesics. Prescription medications may include opioid drugs, such as codeine and morphine, which can lead to addiction. Depending on the particular painkiller, other side effects may include allergic reactions (asthma, swelling, hives, or shock), stomach pains, internal bleeding, heartburn, or nausea. In addition, there may be dangerous interactions between painkillers and other drugs, such as blood thinners or alcohol.

Some chronic pain is so severe that it will necessitate the use of long-term medication. Your physician should be the best guide to such treatment. But be sure when your doctor asks you to list all your medications—a practice that competent caregivers always follow—that you provide a list of everything you're taking, including over-the-counter medications such as aspirin and dietary supplements. To the extent that the chronic pain is exacerbated by stress, mind body techniques, such as those described in the following sections, may be used to decrease the medication.

Scientific Proof for Mind Body Approaches

The scientific literature is replete with support for the use of mind body techniques to counter pains of many types.[58] One of our colleagues, Margaret Caudill, has demonstrated that the relaxation response, in particular, can be a powerful anti-pain treatment.[59]

Another important factor in overcoming pain through a mind body approach is one that we have already discussed in some detail, namely, the placebo effect. To test the efficacy of various anti-pain drugs being considered for the market, researchers use the method known as a "randomized, controlled, double-blind" study. The participants in the experiment are randomly divided into at least two groups, one that receives the drug and the other that receives a placebo pill that looks like the drug but actually is inert. To eliminate outside influences, nobody associated directly with the experiment is told which pill is real and which is the placebo; both participants and physicians are "blind" as to who gets which pill. The objective in setting up a study this way is to try to determine whether a particular drug really can work better than the participant's power of belief—the "placebo effect."

Using this approach in testing painkilling medications, researchers (with informed consent of the participants) have induced pain in the jaws, arms, or other parts of the body. The researchers then administered inert injections or inert pills (placebos), which the participants believed might reduce the pain. The studies have often shown a significant decrease in pain with the placebo, an indication that expectation and belief have the power to counter pain.[60] In fact, the placebos have sometimes caused reduction in perceived pain similar to the pain reduction produced by opioid drugs or other painkillers. Brain scans in participants receiving placebos have revealed significant activity in those parts of the brain involved in the release of opioid pain-relieving neurotransmitters, such as endorphins.[61] Reviews of the medical literature have revealed that hundreds of studies on painkillers have shown that the power of the placebo effect may rival the power of various painkilling drugs.[62]

Similar results have occurred when the impact of surgery on painful conditions was compared with the impact of the placebo effect. In an Australian study reported in the August 6, 2009, issue of the *New England Journal of Medicine*,[63] researchers evaluated the effect of a type of surgery, vertebroplasty, on 71 participants with one or two painful fractures of the vertebrae resulting from osteoporosis (bone-thinning), which were unhealed and had existed less than 12 months.

The researchers emphasize the pervasive nature of this medical problem by noting that about 750,000 new vertebral fractures occur in the United States each year. Also, among people over 50 years of age, up to a quarter will have at least one vertebral fracture in their lifetime. The estimated annual direct-care expenditures for fractures caused by osteoporosis in the United States ranged from $12 billion to $18 billion in 2002, according to an editorial accompanying the article.[64] Vertebroplasty, which involves the injection of a type of cement into the spine at the location of the fracture, has become a common treatment for painful fractures of the vertebrae caused by osteoporosis.

Approximately one-half (35) of the participants in this study were given the actual surgery and the rest (36 participants) received sham surgery, which was designed to appear identical to the real thing. Both study groups experienced "significant reductions" in overall pain, according to a 10-point self-report score. The improvements, which were evaluated three months after the procedures, included reductions in pain at night, at rest, and during physical functioning. The researchers recognized the placebo response to the treatment, which they said might be "amplified" during an invasive treatment such as surgery. They said that "raised expectations of an invasive intervention" may explain the improvements in pain after the sham surgery.[65]

The accompanying editorial in the *New England Journal of Medicine* asked this rhetorical question: "Given the limited effect of vertebroplasty and no significant difference between treatments, was the placebo an active treatment?"

The writer doesn't answer his question directly, though he does say that "compassionate care and tincture of time, in and of themselves, can have an effect." He also says there was evidence in the study of altered fracture healing in the osteoporotic bone, a finding that "might have important implications in the treatment of osteoporotic fracture."[66]

Our answer to the question in the editorial would be more direct: The placebo effect can indeed be an active treatment—and practicing physicians should learn to apply the healing power of expectation-belief, which is associated with the placebo effect, in treating their pain patients.

Possible Mind Body Treatments

Your mind body treatment for pain should include the standard two-phase Benson-Henry Protocol described on page 111.

Because there are many types of pain, which may require different approaches to treatment—especially in the Phase Two visualization—we have included in the following pages some specific suggestions for dealing with these pain variations. In every such variation, Phase One should always be used to calm and open the mind in preparation for the Phase Two visualization. Also, the Phase One relaxation response trigger will itself act directly on the pain through the release of pain-relieving neurotransmitters, such as morphine-like endorphins.

Pain—Variations

Abdominal Pain Visualization

With abdominal pain, your physician must first determine whether there is some organic or physiologic reason for your pain that would require special prescription medications or surgery. Mind body approaches should obviously *not* be regarded as a substitute for standard medical treatment. If you are suffering from an abdominal cancer, other treatments will take a primary role, though mind body approaches may very well be of value in controlling pain.

If your physician cannot identify a particular physical problem that is causing your abdominal pain, a mind body treatment may be in order. Stress-related cramps or abdominal pains often respond quite well to the mind body protocol we recommend.[67]

In employing the Benson-Henry Protocol to relieve your abdominal pain, first evoke the relaxation response in Phase One for 12 to 15 minutes. Then, as you proceed with Phase Two visualization during the last 8 to 10 minutes of the protocol, you might picture yourself sitting quietly watching TV or reading in a state of total relaxation from head to stomach to toe, without any feelings of pain. As you "draw" this mental picture, breathe rhythmically and easily. Steady, unlabored breathing is important for abdominal pain because discomfort in the midsection can be accompanied by a tendency to hold the breath, or even to strain.

What other visualizations might you use for abdominal pain? Because this type of pain often involves cramping and a tendency to "curl up" to relieve the discomfort, see yourself stretched out in complete relaxation on your back, perhaps floating on a lake or reclining on the softest mattress you can imagine. One patient imagined himself floating on a billowing cloud. As you create this mental picture, examine in detail every feature of your environment and your physical responses. What does the cloud look like? How high is it over the earth? Is the lake warm or cool, large or small? Is there a breeze? What are you wearing—if anything? Do your muscles and limbs feel loose and spaghetti-like? If not, focus on those muscles that still seem tight and see them becoming completely relaxed.

Most likely, as you picture yourself in this way, you will experience your abdominal pain at first. That's a normal response. In most cases, those suffering from a particular medical condition find that their discomfort from the condition intensifies when they first focus on it. If this happens, don't stop the visualization exercise. Continue breathing regularly, saying, "Oh well" to the pain.

One reason for the rise of these painful feelings is that as you focus on your body, your mind "remembers" your state of illness and, in effect, reintroduces that remembered pain into your consciousness. But as you picture yourself without the pain, you begin to *remember* what it felt like to be without the pain. Or if you can't quite remember, you at least construct a clear mental picture of what it is like to be without pain. Through this process, remembered wellness gradually replaces remembered illness. Eventually, you may or may not become completely pain free, but you can expect to experience a significant reduction in your pain. If the pain is still there, it will bother you less. You can live with it.

Backache Visualization

Sometimes back pains can signal a serious problem, such as a spinal cord injury, a symptomatic herniated disk (not all herniated disks have symptoms), or a separate illness such as acute pancreatitis or a spinal tumor.[68] Consequently, if your pains persist and you cannot link them to a particular cause such as twisting, lifting, or unusual stress, you should consult with your physician. If you have other symptoms, such as weight loss or pains in other parts of the body, and your backache seems in any way unusual or different from strains and pains you have suffered before, you should definitely contact your physician.

Stress-Related Lower-Back Pain

Often, the common backache, especially in the lower back, may arise from—or be exacerbated by—stress, or by the muscle fatigue and tension caused by stress. Sitting in front of a computer for hours, standing for long periods, or tensing the muscles, including back muscles, when anxious about some family or work situation may trigger a lower-back ache. When the excessive stress is present, a seemingly innocuous act, such as reaching for a cooking utensil or leaning over to brush the teeth, may trigger the pain. Most often, symptoms involve pain around the lower-back "girdle" muscles, running from one side of the lower back to the other.

Mind body relaxation response techniques can be of great help in preventing or treating many types of back pain.[69] An obese patient of mine in her mid-40s, Agnes, developed serious lower-back pain before she came to me, and as a result, she underwent several surgeries. Not only did the surgeries not help her, but her condition grew worse. Her pain levels increased to the point that she could hardly get out of bed in the mornings to get to the law firm where she worked as a secretary. The stresses in her life intensified as she worried about her deteriorating condition and the specter of increased immobility. To be sure, obesity by itself may cause or aggravate a back pain problem. In fact, common medical advice for overweight patients with back problems may be to lose the weight before trying anything else. In Agnes's case, the stress in her life contributed to the pain and had to be confronted medically.

During our first visit, I placed her on a relaxation response treatment plan. As an African-American who came from a strong Christian Gospel tradition, she chose as her focus phrase "peace that passes understanding" from Philippians 4:7. As she repeated this phrase, she quite naturally began to "see" a mental picture of herself in the midst of a bucolic scene with calm pastures and streams. She also saw herself without the back pain. She could actually *remember* what it had felt like a few years previously to be without the pain.

Without any prior planning or direction on my part, she combined her focus phrase (Phase One) with a pleasant, pain-free visualization (Phase Two). Combining the two phases is quite common with some patients, especially among those who are visually oriented. If you find that combining Phases One and Two comes naturally to you—for example, if you automatically see pleasant mental pictures during Phase One—go with it!

After a week or so, Agnes began to feel relief from her pain. In fact, she noticed an improvement after her very first session. She improved so rapidly that she felt confident about accepting an invitation to visit a friend in Uganda. The trip required that she take a plane from Boston to London and then fly to her final destination in Africa. During her visit she was able to walk for several hours at a time and sightsee comfortably with periodic rest periods.

In the past, Agnes had avoided extensive journeys because of her back, but this time she made the entire trip with relatively little pain. Fortunately, Agnes's lower-back pain failed to spread to her buttocks and upper legs, a condition known as sciatica. But Ron wasn't so fortunate.

Referred Back Pain—Sciatica

Sciatica involves pain that typically begins in the lower back and may extend down through the buttocks and into the back of the upper leg.

In the most severe cases, the pains may reach down into the lower leg and foot. The cause of this pain may be a herniated disk, an infection, a tumor, or stress.[70] If your physician determines that the cause of your problem is probably stress—or that stress is likely a component of the complaint—a mind body approach is in order.

Ron developed a debilitating lower-back pain while he was brushing his teeth one morning, a simple activity that seemed too harmless to cause the pain. Yet the back pain persisted, and within a week severe sciatic pain began shooting from his lower left back, through his left buttock, and down into his left leg. He also started to feel a tingling in his left foot.

Discussions during his first medical examination revealed the probable underlying triggers for the condition: He had recently undergone several high-stress challenges in his life, including a divorce and a move to another part of town. Also, his personal pressures were exacerbating the normal stress he felt at work. His physicians determined that he was already under considerable stress and the tooth brushing had merely triggered the pain.

As a result of this diagnosis, Ron was referred to a counselor who was experienced in mind body treatments. This expert bolstered Ron's belief in the efficacy of a mind body approach by referring him to the scientific literature. Among other things, the counselor explained how the relaxation response, combined with appropriate visualizations, could produce healing by changing his various physiologic reactions, including a lowered metabolism and decreased blood pressure.

The counselor then taught Ron how to elicit the relaxation response, using the basic eight-step procedure summarized on page 111. Ron found that it took him about nine minutes to settle down mentally and become immersed in subjective feelings of inner calm and relaxation, and he usually continued in this state for another five minutes. The counselor also showed Ron how to include healing visualizations in his treatment. Among other things, he encouraged Ron to conceive a mental picture of what it had been like to walk and move about without the sciatica. Ron would contemplate this scene for about 8 to 10 minutes during Phase Two of the Benson-Henry Protocol. Through the visualization he found a way to "remember" a prior state of wellness, which he hoped to recapture.

After a few days of pursuing this daily treatment plan, Ron noticed that the pains in his lower leg and back had mostly disappeared. He still felt some stiffness in his lower back, but that discomfort did not prevent him from moving about with relative freedom. Before two weeks had elapsed, he even planned a short holiday at a nearby resort, a possibility that he would not have considered when he was in severe back and sciatic pain.

What happened inside Ron could be explained scientifically this way:

Most likely, the extra stress in his life had turned on gene activity that led to muscle spasms and pain. Ron's brain, nerves, and muscles had been "rewired" to feel pain. Through the mechanism known as neuroplasticity, pain stimulated by some outside factor such as stress may cause the brain to reorganize itself by establishing new neural connections through nerve cells (neurons).[71] This reorganization produced and sustained Ron's pain. Even when some of the stressors bearing down on Ron had subsided, including the worries surrounding his divorce, the rewired areas continued stimulating the pain. Ron needed an outside influence or force to "remold" his plastic brain into a "pain-free shape."

When he began eliciting the Phase One relaxation response, Ron "switched on" anti-stress gene activity, which caused various parts of his body to work against the pain. Also, as he visualized freedom from pain—in other words, as he recaptured a state of remembered wellness without physical discomfort—he began to develop an inner expectation-belief that he really possessed the inherent capacity to counter the pain. With the further help of this placebo-effect factor, his physiology, including brain responses, nerves, and hormones, was rewired once more to enable him to return to a relatively pain-free condition.

Headache Visualization

Some headaches—such as those accompanied by a high fever, blurred vision, vomiting, or mental confusion—require immediate medical attention. A concussion, meningitis, encephalitis, or brain hemorrhage may be responsible for these symptoms. If you experience such a headache, you should consult a physician immediately. Other headaches—such as tension, migraine, and cluster headaches—may respond well to painkillers and/or mind body techniques.[72]

The "Mind Body Headaches"

- *Tension headaches.* Although the cause is unknown, the symptoms typically include a sense of tightness, as though a circular band is being squeezed around the head. The pain, which frequently begins late in the day, may last for varying lengths of time and may recur on a regular basis. Physicians often prescribe painkillers or recommend over-the-counter drugs such as aspirin. This condition may respond well to stress management procedures (see below).

- *Migraine headaches.* Migraines involve a throbbing pain that may start in one part of the head and spread to other parts. Other symptoms may include "down" feelings, fatigue, loss of appetite, or visual responses such as a sense of seeing flashing lights. Treatments and preventive measures include avoiding environments that may produce migraines (such as those with certain lights or odors). Some prescription medicines, such as beta-blockers, aspirin, or antidepressants, may help. Mind body treatments have also worked well with many people (see below).

- *Cluster headaches.* Sharp pains in a particular eye several times each day characterize these headaches. Many times, they begin after the patient falls asleep. Aspirin, other over-the-counter drugs, or prescribed painkillers may be recommended. Physicians may prescribe inhaling oxygen for those cluster headaches that arise mainly at night. In addition, mind body approaches may be of help, especially when combined with other medical procedures (see below).

Scientific Support for Mind Body Treatments for Headaches

Tension, migraine, and cluster headaches often respond well to mind body techniques. In the very first clinical study I conducted in 1974, I collaborated with John R. Graham of Harvard Medical School in evaluating 17 patients suffering from migraine headache and four from cluster headache.[73]

Each of the 21 patients in the study had a long history of severe pains, a history of drug therapy, and little relief from symptoms. After at least four months of eliciting the relaxation response, using an approach that was consistent with our basic Phase One template, six of the 17 migraine patients experienced improvement in their symptoms, with four becoming virtually headache free. Of the four cluster headache patients, one had a "remarkable" clinical headache recovery that lasted longer than a year. Two of the other cluster headache patients showed improvement for several months but then lapsed back into their previous headache patterns.

The intriguing results of this initial study prompted me to do a number of subsequent investigations into the impact of mind body treatments on headaches, with highly encouraging results. Our studies to date have shown that about 60 percent of patients with migraine headaches experience fewer and less severe headaches after they use relaxation response techniques.[74] In another study, more than one-third of the patients, including many with head pains, reduced their visits to physicians to treat the pain.[75]

In 2009, we conducted a study of 640 outpatients who underwent a 12-week mind body medical symptom reduction program at the Mind/Body Medical Institute in Boston. Patients with headaches experienced a significant reduction in pre-treatment versus post-treatment headaches. The headache frequency declined to an average of less than twice a month from an average of several times a month.[76]

A number of studies have established that relief from chronic headache syndromes, such as tension and migraine, is possible for patients who use either the basic relaxation response trigger, which utilizes a focus word or phrase, or progressive relaxation. You'll recall that we recommend a short progressive relaxation exercise be used at the beginning of the relaxation response elicitation. This procedure involves tensing and then relaxing muscles progressively throughout the body, beginning with the toes and ending with the shoulders and head. Other studies have shown that using such a progressive relaxation exercise *throughout* Phase One is effective for eliciting the relaxation response and also for healing of conditions such as chronic headaches.[77]

Headache Visualizations

Our studies show that just eliciting the relaxation response by itself is often enough to relieve or cure a chronic headache. But because other studies have established that the placebo effect is also a highly effective mind body treatment for pain, we strongly recommend that you include the expectation-belief dimension of Phase Two visualization as part of your plan to counter your headaches.

For example, after you spend about 15 minutes eliciting the relaxation response in Phase One, you might sit quietly, with eyes closed, and picture yourself engaging in some favorite activity—without any headache. Although you don't want to focus on the pain, you might select a scene that typically triggers a headache. Some patients may choose to see themselves reading a book. Others may visualize their participation in an athletic activity or a family holiday dinner. Whatever scene you choose, try to reach back into your memories to recall a time of remembered wellness when you could engage in your chosen activity without any headache.

Caution: It is almost certain that when you begin this visualization exercise, you will at some point experience a headache. Don't let the pain deter you from sticking with your mental picture for the prescribed 8 to 10 minutes. To make the process easier for yourself, try turning away from the pain with a silent "Oh well"—just as you would do during the Phase One triggering of the relaxation response.

Or you might actually *welcome* the onset of the headache. Say something like this to the pain: "Hi there! I expected you to join me. Okay, let's enter this scene together at the family dinner table, or with a good book, or wherever. But I do expect you to tire of this activity at some point and leave me alone—and that will be okay, too." By establishing such a playful conversation with your pain, you will affirm that there is something powerful within you that can help control the pain and objectify it.

Don't try to fight the headache. Just allow it to come and go as it "wills." You will gradually become desensitized to the pain, the frequency of onset will decrease, and the episodes will eventually disappear.

Migraines in Children

The elicitation of the relaxation response can also be effective in the treatment of migraines among children. In a randomized, controlled investigation conducted at Children's Hospital Boston, under the leadership of David Fentress of Children's Hospital and Harvard Medical School, we studied 18 children ages eight to 12 who were suffering from migraine headaches.[78]

Requirements to participate in the study included neurological tests to confirm the migraine diagnosis. The subjects needed to be suffering from at least three severe headache symptoms, such as throbbing pain, nausea, pain during movement, or certain phobias, including fears of light or odors. Patients in the study also had to have suffered from at least three headaches during the past month, but they could not suffer constantly from headaches or headache-related symptoms.

We devoted the first four weeks of the study to assessing the headache occurrences in the children. Then, we set aside nine weeks for training groups of children in mind body techniques.

Six of the children in the study received a relaxation response training period and also instruction in pain behavior management. The training included the main features of the basic relaxation response trigger that we teach as Phase One of the Benson-Henry Protocol. The children's individual relaxation response sessions, where they focused on breathing and a focus word or phrase, were limited to about 10 minutes.

Six of the other children received training with biofeedback devices and with the two treatments used by the first group (training in relaxation response elicitation and pain behavior management). The biofeedback device involved the placement of electrodes on the children's foreheads and a temperature sensor on the middle finger of their dominant hand. With these procedures, we were able to monitor their brain waves and other physiologic responses. The final six children constituted a control group with no special training. All participants kept records of their headaches during the 15-week study period and also for four weeks at the end of the study. The children's parents helped with the reporting.

The results confirmed that migraine headaches in children were one more medical condition that responded well to mind body treatments. Both treatment groups experienced a significant reduction in headache symptoms as compared to the control group. Both treatment groups enjoyed about the same level of improvement, and the effects were long-lasting: The treatment groups maintained their reduction in headache symptoms one year after treatment ended.

We concluded in our study: "These results suggest that relaxation response training, with or without biofeedback training, combined with pain behavior management, is an effective alternative treatment for pediatric migraine."

How Children with Headaches Can Visualize

A mother came to my office with her eight-year-old son, who had been diagnosed with congenital migraine headaches. As an infant, he had cried much more than the average child. The parents didn't know the reason until he got old enough to verbalize that he had headaches.

His pediatrician eventually diagnosed the boy's condition as congenital migraine headaches, or migraines since birth. Because of the frequency and severity of the attacks, he missed a lot of school in his elementary years and fell several grades behind his age group. The intensity of the headaches forced him to retreat into a darkened room, where he would just wait them out. Although the boy tried a variety of medications, none worked to significantly reduce the severity of the headaches.

Learning that the family members were strong Roman Catholics and that the child was being brought up in Roman Catholicism, I suggested that he choose "Hail Mary, full of grace" as his focus phrase as he practiced Phase One of our protocol. The repetition of these comforting words helped him trigger the relaxation response more readily.

Repeating words rooted in his religious faith also prepared him to move easily into Phase Two visualizations: Thinking of the Virgin Mary enhanced his ability to "draw" a positive mental picture that was conducive to healing. Finally, I suggested that he begin to say the rosary when the warning signals (the prodrome) of the migraine started. His particular warning signals included an increased sense of fatigue and a greater sensitivity to light.

Shortly after the boy started this mind body treatment regimen, the intensity of the headaches subsided. Within weeks, he found that he could actually abort the headaches just after they started or even prevent them from developing after the prodrome stage. Before long, he returned to school and caught up quickly with his studies and his proper grade.

Joint Pain Visualization

Pain in the joints, including pain resulting from rheumatoid arthritis, can often be alleviated by strong expectation or belief that a certain treatment will succeed, according to several studies focusing on the placebo effect. One study established that 40 percent of patients receiving placebos have experienced a 50 percent reduction in the number of swollen joints and a 50 percent reduction in joint swelling and tenderness. The relief from pain and swelling lasted at least six months.[79]

How might you foster such belief inside yourself—and increase your own chances of mitigating rheumatoid arthritis symptoms?

Assume you have rheumatoid arthritis in your fingers, with pain, swelling, and stiffness. After evoking the relaxation response in Phase One of your mind body treatment, begin Phase Two with a slow-motion visualization of yourself rotating, stretching, or otherwise using those finger joints that give you the most discomfort.

During Phase One, you have already gone through a preliminary muscle-relaxing exercise, which involved focusing on relaxing each part of your body, including your arms, hands, and fingers. Now, return your focus to your hands. Breathe slowly and regularly, with your eyes closed. Without actually moving anything, picture yourself slowly flexing and extending the fingers of your right hand. Continue with this image for four or five minutes. Now see yourself executing the same movements with your left fingers and hand for the same length of time.

If you sense any pain as you think of these movements, don't become concerned. Remember that it's quite natural to experience the very symptom you want to eliminate when you first begin your visualization. That's a natural part of the healing process. But you can expect, if you continue with the visualizations over a period of days, that healing and a lessening of the pain will occur. Throughout, continue to breathe deeply and rhythmically.

As you proceed with these visualizations in later weeks, you may want to vary the mental pictures of your movements. There are a couple of reasons for this approach. For one thing, seeing the same image over and over may become tedious and could encourage a tendency to skip the exercise rather than become bored. In addition, visualizing yourself in a variety of different situations may help promote the healing process. Assume that you have created a mental image of yourself lifting a bag of groceries without pain or stiffness, even though you are using an arthritic hand. Focus on that image during Phase Two over a period of days or weeks. Most likely, when you confront the actual challenge of *physically* lifting groceries, you will be able to do so with lessened pain or even no pain.

Knee Pain Visualization

Some knee pains are clearly the result of trauma or other health problems that require direct intervention using conventional medical treatments, such as drugs or surgery. If you bump or twist your knee during athletic activity and then experience tenderness, swelling, or bruising, it is highly likely that the injury or activity is the cause of your problem. A fracture, dislocation, or torn ligament will require standard medical follow-up, such as a painkilling medication or surgery. Or your physician may prescribe the familiar RICE treatment for recovery: rest, ice application, compression, and elevation to prevent swelling.[80]

On the other hand, some recent research suggests that with some knee pain, mind body treatments may play a significant role.

The Mind Body Option

On page 72 of Chapter 5, we introduced an important 2002 study published in the *New England Journal of Medicine,* which explored the link between knee pain and the placebo effect. This report suggested that with some knee pain, belief and expectation in the likelihood of healing may be as effective a treatment as arthroscopic surgery.[81] To reinforce your own understanding of—and belief in—this research, it will be helpful to examine that investigation more closely.

Baylor College of Medicine scientists studied 180 individuals with osteoarthritis (wear-and-tear arthritis) of the knee, 165 of whom completed the experiment. Participants were randomly assigned to receive one of three treatments: 1) arthroscopic* debridement (removal of dead tissue inside the knee); 2) arthroscopic lavage (washing-out of the knee joint); or 3) placebo "sham" surgery. All patients and assessors of the study outcome were "blinded" as to which patients got the real treatments and which received the placebo. The researchers assessed the outcomes of the procedures over a 24-month period with the use

---

* Arthroscopy refers to the use of an arthroscope, usually a fiber-optic instrument inserted through a small incision near a joint, such as the knee joint, to permit observation of the inside of the joint. Surgical procedures can then be performed through the arthroscope.

of five self-reported scores for pain and physical function. The participants also engaged in one objective test of walking and stair climbing.

The results were rather startling. The researchers reported that at no point did the arthroscopic-intervention groups—the patients who had received the real surgery—have less knee pain or better function than the placebo group. The sham surgery worked as well as the real thing. The researchers concluded there was no clinically meaningful difference between the groups. At some points during follow-up, objective physical function of the patients was significantly *worse* in the surgical group than in the placebo group!

The researchers further observed that this lack of difference in the results suggested that the improvement was not due to any intrinsic efficacy of the procedures. Rather, the most powerful factor in improvement might have been the natural healing history of the medical condition or an independent effect of the placebo—that is, the belief and expectation on the part of the patients that the procedure would work.

Finally, the authors of the study put a price tag on their findings. They noted that if the value of real arthroscopic surgery in patients with osteoarthritis of the knee is no greater than that of "sham" placebo surgery, then "the billions of dollars spent on such procedures annually might be put to better use." In any case, they said, health-care researchers should not underestimate the power of the placebo effect.

Researchers from the Department of Orthopedic Surgery, University of Pennsylvania, reviewed and endorsed the validity of this study the following year. They confirmed that the data presented in the *New England Journal of Medicine* report suggest that the benefit of arthroscopy for the treatment of osteoarthritis of the knee is to provide subjective pain relief, and that the means by which arthroscopy provides this benefit is the placebo effect.[82]

Visualization Suggestions

This study strongly suggests that many arthroscopic surgeries to relieve knee pain from osteoarthritis may work simply because the patient believes and expects that the procedure will work. So how might you capture this power of belief and expectation if you are wrestling with this type of knee pain?

Obviously, you do not have the benefit of being in a well-controlled study involving such procedures as sham surgery. But by *accepting* and *believing* the validity of such investigations as this one and also by employing the type of visualization that we are recommending— visualization coupled with your own belief system—you will be in a strong position to replicate the placebo effect that produced the knee pain relief in this particular study.

Here is a suggestion for appropriating the power of expectation- belief to alleviate your pain:

First, proceed through Phase One, the evocation of the relaxation response for the recommended 12 to 15 minutes. Now, with your physiologic and genetic activity working to enhance the power of your personal belief systems, proceed with Phase Two of the protocol: Take 8 to 10 minutes to contemplate your hurting knee. Keep your eyes closed, breathe regularly, and don't move the knee physically or even in your mind's eye. Just use your mind to "watch" the resting knee. Examine it from all angles.

As you visualize, reach back in time to a point when your knee was completely well, free of all pain. You might think, "That's a pretty good knee. It really works well. I can perform all sorts of physical feats using that knee."

Very slowly, see yourself raising your knee and leg off the ground. Again, you feel no discomfort or pain. Or if pain enters when you begin to think this way, just say, "Come on in. You're not so bad. And I know you won't last. You can't outlast me and my healing mental movie."

Continue to see your knee move about with no feelings of pain. Again, if the pain creeps in, think, "That pain doesn't belong in this scene. That's pain that came along later. I'm in a time past, when there was no pain."

Always remember that feeling some pain during these visualiza- tions is part of the healing process. It's quite natural to sense some pain right at the beginning of the Phase Two exercise. But you can also be confident that the pain will subside and disappear—just as it did with the participants in the *New England Journal of Medicine* study.

Neck and Shoulder Pain Visualization

Neck pain, including pains that extend from the neck into the shoulders, may result from a medical condition such as a spinal cord injury, a whiplash injury, meningitis, a hemorrhage, strep throat, or cancer of the lymph glands. But more often, the neck pains arise from fatigue- or stress-related situations that can be countered with appropriate mind body treatments. Remember that even if the pain comes from a serious health problem, mind body approaches may help mitigate the pain, along with other medical measures.[83]

In a study conducted through the Harvard Medical School under the leadership of Margaret Caudill, we evaluated 109 patients with assorted pains, including 19 with neck pain. They were participating in an outpatient behavioral medicine program at the Matthew Thornton Health Plan, an HMO in Nashua, New Hampshire.[84] To evaluate the impact of the mind body techniques used, including the elicitation of the relaxation response, we focused on data showing the extent to which the participants returned to work or to further treatment at the medical clinic. Returning to work would indicate improvement, while returning to the clinic would point to ongoing pain.

Using these criteria, we found a decided level of improvement in patients who followed the mind body regimen, which featured the relaxation response. A 36 percent reduction in clinic visits resulted in the first year after the mind body intervention. Also, the decreased clinic use continued among the first 50 patients who were followed for two years after the intervention.

What Causes the Stress-Related Neck Pain?

Many times, stress-related pains in the arms or shoulders may appear as a result of cramped working positions, cramped sleeping positions, old injuries, a sedentary lifestyle, stiffness from aging, or a variety of other factors. Even when the obvious cause of the pain has been remedied, such as by your working or sleeping in a more comfortable position or embarking on an exercise program to relax and strengthen sore muscles, the pain lingers. These pain signals from the brain to the body often remain strong, as a kind of "phantom pain." (You'll recall that when a limb is amputated, the amputee may still experience feelings, including these "phantom pains," in the missing body part.) In such cases, even though the source of pain has been eliminated, the negatively rewired sections of the brain and nervous system continue to "remember the pain."

The Secret of Successful of Mind Body Treatment

To overcome these painful perceptions, you might use a visualization exercise that utilizes remembered wellness about a time when you were without pain in your neck or shoulder. Begin your mind body treatment as usual with the Phase One elicitation of the relaxation response. Then, as you move into the Phase Two visualizations, allow your memories to drift back weeks, months, or years to a time when you could sit or move without the pain. Recall a specific instance when you were painless. Possibilities include a particularly relaxing vacation or holiday or a pleasant outing with a child or other family member.

Simply evoking the relaxation response in Phase One may be enough to eliminate your neck pain. But if you combine these Phase Two visualization suggestions with your Phase One approach, it is likely that you will increase your chances of replacing your remembered pain with remembered wellness.

Visualization to Prepare for Surgical Distress

Surgery of any type is often followed by pain. In addition, both before and after surgery patients may experience signs of emotional or physiological distress, such as anxiety, anger, or an unusually fast heart rate. Known as tachycardia, this last condition may involve a heart rate of 100 beats to the minute or more.

Typically, surgeons will prescribe only painkillers, tranquilizers, or other medications to minimize these effects. But many times, mind body techniques can be employed with other medical measures to reduce uncomfortable pre- and postoperative physical and psychological reactions to surgery.

A Case of Cardiac Surgery

In a 1989 study published in *Behavioral Medicine,* under the leadership of Jane Leserman of our Institute, we evaluated 27 cardiac bypass surgery patients who were randomly assigned to one of two groups, one experimental and the other control.[85] The experimental group, consisting of 13 patients, received educational information before the surgery and also practiced eliciting the relaxation response before and after surgery. The 14 patients in the control group received only the educational information.

Those who practiced the relaxation response technique received their mind body training two to seven days before their surgery and were asked to practice the technique both before and after the surgery. They were also given a relaxation response tape that led them through a modified progressive muscle relaxation exercise. Even with their rather minimal level of mind body training, the experimental group experienced several beneficial results.

First of all, they had a lower incidence of postoperative rapid heartbeats (supraventricular tachycardia) than did the control group. They also experienced greater decreases in psychological tension. (The authors of the study qualified this finding in one respect: They noted that the decreases in tension in the experimental group may have been more dramatic because that group, as a result of the random selection, started the study at a higher level of tension than did the control group.) Additionally, the experimental group had reduced levels of anger in comparison with the control group.

The Mind and Skin Cancer

In another investigation published in the *Journal of Human Stress* and led by Alice Domar of Beth Israel Deaconess Medical Center and Harvard Medical School, we studied 42 patients who received skin cancer surgery for melanoma and for less serious basal-cell and squamous-cell skin cancers.[86] The participating patients were divided into a control and an experimental group.

The control group of 21 patients read material of their choice daily for 20 minutes for an average of 27 days before surgery. The experimental group of 21 patients was trained in how to evoke the relaxation response and did so for at least 20 minutes each day. They followed this procedure for an average of 24 days before their surgery. To assist them with the relaxation response exercise (Phase One of our Benson-Henry Protocol), we provided the members of the experimental group with three aids: 1) a cassette tape that gave step-by-step instructions in eliciting the response; 2) a one-page instruction sheet; and 3) a chapter from my first book, *The Relaxation Response*. Both the control and the experimental groups were given daily diary sheets and instructed to report on their emotional and physical responses.

A limit on the applicability of this study was the relatively minor nature of much of the skin surgery that was performed. But we did find statistically significant subjective differences in the two groups: Those in the experimental group, who had used the relaxation response technique, said that the technique had reduced their anxiety several days before surgery. Their highest levels of anxiety occurred prior to their joining the study. The control group, in contrast, experienced their highest levels of anxiety during and after surgery. We concluded that regular elicitation of the relaxation response can alter subjective reports of distress or anxiety associated with surgery.

The use of mind body techniques to minimize pre- and postoperative discomfort experienced by patients remains a research work-in-progress. Our studies suggest that employing Phase One, the triggering of the relaxation response, has considerable potential for eliminating anxiety or fear during or after surgery, if not actual pain. But there are also some indications in the research that utilization of the visualization techniques in Phase Two can be helpful.

One clinical example of the power of Phase Two mental imagery involved a patient with skin cancer who had been trained in relaxation response and visualization techniques. This patient, Carl, had actually studied the medical reports on using mind body techniques with surgical procedures, which you are reading in this book. He had also practiced the two-phase technique for several months before he confronted his medical problem.

Carl had been diagnosed through a biopsy as having a small basal-cell cancer on his cheek, which required several rather painful injections of local anesthesia to numb the area of the operation. The cancer was surgically removed, and the wound was cauterized and sutured. The medical procedures included measuring the patient's blood pressure before and after the operation.

Using our recommended method of eliciting the relaxation response before, during, and after outpatient surgery, Carl repeated slowly the first lines of the 23rd Psalm in the traditional King James Version of the Bible: "The Lord is my shepherd, I shall not want. He maketh me to lie down in green pastures: he leadeth me beside the still waters. He restoreth my soul. . . ." Simultaneously, he "drew" a mental picture of peaceful green pastures and still waters. As the surgery proceeded, he switched his mind body technique to a focus that involved slowly counting backward from the number 25 and then repeating the backward count if necessary. He had no anxious feelings throughout the procedure.

During the first blood-pressure measurement as he lay on the operating platform before the surgery began, Carl's readings were 126/70 mm Hg, or sufficiently low under the stressful circumstances to prompt the attending nurse to exclaim, "My, you have low blood pressure!" The readings were lower than he usually had during other medical examinations. He recalled that the mental images he had employed of "green pastures" and "still waters" had overshadowed thoughts of the surgery he was undergoing.

After the surgery, Carl's systolic blood-pressure reading had risen slightly to 132 mm Hg, but his diastolic had decreased to 68 mm Hg.

The surgeon and nurse both noted that the local anesthesia contained ingredients that tended to raise blood pressure slightly. Hours after the surgery, after the numbing effects of the anesthesia had worn off, he experienced almost no pain except for a slight aching in his cheek. Although in a similar, previous skin surgery he had required repeated doses of oral painkillers to help him "stay ahead of the pain," in this case he required no painkillers at all.

In this particular case, several factors appear to have been in play:

First, Carl had elicited the Phase One changes associated with the relaxation response—changes that have been linked to lower anxiety levels and lower blood pressure.

Second, his description of his Phase Two visualization indicates that he had engaged some of his deepest beliefs on several levels. For one thing, he had recently studied and *believed* the scientific literature showing that mind body approaches can have significant health benefits in surgical procedures. Also, he made use of his spiritual beliefs by relying on a passage of Old Testament Scripture or other spiritual imagery before, during, and after the surgery. He reported that the visualizations seemed to overpower the anxious and painful feelings he had previously associated with this kind of outpatient surgery.

Finally, Carl had become experienced in the months before his surgery in using our two-phase mind body protocol. He had employed these techniques frequently enough to become confident that they would work in a medical setting.

Guided Imagery in Italy

Further scientific support for the power of using Phase Two visualization with surgery may be found in a 2000 study published in the *International Journal of Colorectal Diseases*. This investigation evaluated the use of guided imagery in dealing with pain and other discomforts associated with rectal and anal surgery.[87]

The Italian investigators divided the 86 patients into one group of 43 who received standard proctological and surgical care, and an experimental group of 43 who employed relaxation techniques. The relaxation group participants listened to a tape that guided them through a series of pleasant, calm mental images—with soothing music and audio text—before, during, and after their surgery.

The researchers established three criteria to evaluate whether or not the relaxation technique worked: 1) postoperative pain experienced by each patient, as measured by a standard self-reported score; 2) the quality of the patient's sleep, as measured by a similar score; and 3) the nature of first urination of each patient, which would be evaluated as "normal" or "difficult."

The researchers found that patients using the relaxation technique with the guided imagery exercise experienced a reduction of pain following the surgery, a significant improvement in the quality of sleep, and a decrease in anxiety. They recommended the use of guided imagery, "a low cost and noninvasive procedure," as a helpful tool in this type of surgery.

Further Implications for Your Visualizations

These studies suggest several possibilities for surgical patients who are exploring the use of mind body visualization to prepare themselves for their operation:

In the first place, our Phase One relaxation response will be likely to reduce the negative physical effects of anxiety, fear, or other negative emotions in most patients facing serious surgery. Also, Phase One can be used to open the patient's mind to receive positive facts and expectations about the probable success of the surgery. With the mind open to positive suggestion and information, Phase Two visualization will also help the patient process the facts that suggest surgery is the right path to follow. This Phase Two exercise will implant the idea that the surgery will probably be successful and lead to healing.

Note: A major objective of both the Phase One and Phase Two components of this mind body treatment is to get the surgery patient's conscious mind to focus on nonstressful mental images and thoughts *to the exclusion of specific thoughts about the surgery.* In a previous publication, we cited an example of how very psychotic patients may do better than mentally healthy patients in recovering from surgery.[88] Because the attention of mentally challenged patients can often be diverted from other matters, including a pending medical procedure, they may be less likely to experience undue anxiety and other negative emotional side effects associated with a serious operation.

So how might these principles work in practice? Here is how you might apply the two-phase protocol when you face surgery that requires general anesthesia:

First, well in advance of the surgical procedure, begin your mind body preparation. On a daily basis, you should assume a comfortable position in a quiet place, close your eyes, and proceed for 12 to 15 minutes with the Phase One relaxation response trigger.

Next, with your eyes closed for the 8 to 10 minutes of Phase Two visualization, create a pleasant mental scene. Because this surgery will require that you be unconscious with general anesthesia, you might see yourself getting pleasantly drowsy and then going to sleep. Then picture yourself waking up with the operation completely finished! (You should not try to imagine what is going on in the operating room while you're asleep. After all, that won't be a direct part of your personal experience because you won't be aware of anything.) In the last scene of your mental movie, see yourself completely healed, participating in all sorts of vigorous activities.

If you have initial fears and anxieties about undergoing serious surgery or about facing an extended period of recuperation, that is quite natural. Everyone—including physicians—has the same feelings. But the more you can "see" how you are likely to experience a complete recovery, the more deconditioned or desensitized you will become to the normal fears and anxieties. Negative emotions, such as anxiety, can contribute to many types of postoperative discomfort, including pain. But controlling the negative emotions could help you recover quite successfully.

Parkinson's Disease

Symptoms

Typically a condition that afflicts both men and women 55 and older, Parkinson's disease is caused by the death of nerve cells and the loss of the neurotransmitter dopamine.

Symptoms may include increasing rigidity of muscles, slowness of physical movement (bradykinesia), trembling of hands, walking characterized by small steps and loss of balance, sleep problems, and difficulties in swallowing and speaking. Eventually, some form of dementia affects up to 20 percent of those with this disease.[89]

Standard Medical Treatments

Although there is no cure for this disease, certain medicines, usually both levodopa (L-dopa) and carbidopa, may help to produce needed dopamine and relieve symptoms. But after about five years, the effect of the drugs tends to diminish.[90] Side effects may include a return of intensified Parkinson's symptoms, such as being physically "frozen" or unable to move, and also psychotic episodes.

In addition to drugs, some forms of surgery may be helpful. For example, with procedures such as pallidotomy or thalamotomy the surgeon destroys a small part of the brain. These procedures can relieve rigidity, slowness of movement, and trembling in more than 90 percent of patients.[91] Efforts are also under way to develop other types of surgery.

Scientific Proof for Mind Body Approaches

Because standard treatments for Parkinson's, such as drugs, have side effects or provide relatively short-term relief, interest has increased in the use of mind body approaches that may work alone or with drugs or surgery. In particular, as discussed on page 85 in Chapter 5, the landmark Fuente-Fernández study[92] established the power of the placebo effect as a means to generate dopamine and help combat Parkinson's disease. In that investigation, the researchers introduced the placebo effect by having the patients take inert pills rather than levodopa medication. They found that the placebo pills caused the patients to produce the neurotransmitter dopamine, which is deficient in Parkinson's. In some instances, the placebo worked better than the actual medication. Later studies and review articles have supported the findings that *expectation* of improvement or cure by a Parkinson's patient can actually improve motor movement.[93]

The power of expectation-belief has also been effective in studies evaluating the use of surgery. In 2004 in the *Archives of General Psychiatry,*[94] researchers compared the responses of one group of Parkinson's patients, who underwent a transplant of human embryonic dopamine neurons into the brain, with a second group who received a form of sham surgery. This investigation was designed as a double-blind study, with none of the parties or researchers being aware of which participants were getting the real or sham treatment. The researchers found that those who *believed* that they had received the transplants—even if they hadn't—not only produced increased levels of dopamine but also reported better scores on "quality of life" measurements and improvement in their physical symptoms.

A major limitation of these surgery studies is similar to the limitation of drugs used to treat Parkinson's: The benefits of the placebo effect have been only short-term. The possible longer-term value of expectation-belief remains to be explored in later studies.

Possible Mind Body Treatments

An effective mind body treatment to counter Parkinson's disease should include the basic two-phase Benson-Henry Protocol summarized on page 111.

Because the placebo effect—the expectation and belief of the patient in the possibility of healing—has been so important in Parkinson's research, we recommend that you place particular emphasis on visualizing yourself in a vigorous, healthy condition in Phase Two. To find a rich mental image that will occupy you for a longer period, you may have to spend a little more time preparing for the exercise.

Think back a few years and remember those times when you were in excellent health. You might try this memory exercise:

Think about yourself in a particular situation that you can actually recall, say, approximately two years ago. Perhaps the situation involved a family holiday or a weekend sports outing. You should be able to remember yourself walking and moving with quick, agile physical movements, unimpeded by your present physical rigidity and bradykinesia, or slowness of movement. If your Parkinson's disease symptoms have lasted longer than two years, then go back five years, or seven, or however long a period is necessary to see yourself well, active, and vigorous.

In searching for a real past scene in which you were symptom free, you may have to ask for help from a friend or family member. Or maybe you can consult a journal you keep or an old scheduling book. When you have the incident in mind, contemplate it. Recall the people you were with and what you did together. Settle upon a particularly satisfying scene or perhaps a couple of scenes and savor them for a while. You'll be surprised how quickly the time will pass as you immerse yourself in that past event. Return to these remembered scenes for 8 to 10 minutes each day as you practice Phase Two of your mind body protocol.

By focusing on Phase Two visualization in this way, you will be more likely to generate a level of expectation-belief that could produce healing forces similar to those unleashed by the placebo effect in the Fuente-Fernández study. At the same time, you will be using a technique that will counter harmful feelings of stress that may accompany your condition and threaten your health in other ways.

Phobias

Symptoms

A phobia is an extremely strong, illogical, and recurrent fear that tends to be triggered when the person is in a certain situation or encounter. The fear is typically not rational because the situation or object of the fear may pose no real threat. But the emotional response can quickly turn into uncontrollable terror, with the shortness of breath, pounding heart, and other symptoms characteristic of high anxiety or a panic attack. An estimated 5 to 13 percent of Americans of all ages suffer from such phobias. Population groups that tend to suffer most from phobias include women and men over the age of 25.[95]

Although psychologists and psychiatrists have compiled lists that run on for pages, some of the most common phobias include claustrophobia (fear of closed spaces or confinement), agoraphobia (fear of open or public places), ochlophobia (fear of crowds), acrophobia (fear of heights), taphophobia (fear of being buried alive), cynophobia (fear of dogs), astrapophobia (fear of lightning), keraunophobia (fear of thunder), acousticophobia or phonophobia (fear of sounds), photophobia (fear of light), ophidiophobia (fear of snakes), arachnophobia (fear of spiders), laliophobia (fear of speaking), hemophobia (fear of blood), xenophobia (fear of strangers), theophobia (fear of God), and vaccinophobia (fear of vaccination).

Standard Medical Treatments

One approach to treatment of phobias involves medications.[96] Selective serotonin reuptake inhibitors (SSRIs), antidepressants that increase levels of the hormone serotonin, may be prescribed. But SSRIs may interact with other drugs, such as anticonvulsants, antihistamines, or other antidepressants and may, depending on the drug and the patient, cause dizziness, nausea, heart rate abnormalities, or even death. Monoamine oxidase inhibitors (MAOI), another drug remedy for phobias, may have emotional side effects, such as altered consciousness. Physicians may also prescribe beta-blockers (possible side effect: drowsiness) or the sedative abenzodiazepine (possible side effect: drowsiness). These and other drugs may lead to dependence or may actually increase anxieties, depending on individual patient reactions.

Although some medications may help some patients on a temporary basis, the preferred treatments lie in the mind body area. The most effective include *relaxation therapy* of the type we are recommending in this book and *desensitization therapy*. With desensitization therapy, the patient is typically exposed to the feared object or situation, either in incremental doses over a period of time or all at once. Studies and clinical observations have established that the more familiar and less sensitive a patient becomes when encountering a feared entity or computerized images that simulate the feared entity,[97] the more likely is it that the phobia will disappear. Once the therapy has succeeded, the patient usually is free of the phobia permanently.[98]

Scientific Proof for Mind Body Approaches

A consensus is emerging in the scientific literature that the best way to treat most phobias is to use a two-pronged approach: 1) a desensitization procedure involving actual or "virtual" exposure (usually through computer imaging) to the feared situation or object, and 2) relaxation therapy.

Our studies clearly show that the relaxation response triggers physiologic reactions that are associated with altered autonomic nervous system activity—changes in the body that help counter the anxiety symptoms associated with a phobic reaction. Also, the relaxation response produces a mental calming that helps the phobic patient focus attention on the object of desensitization. This increased ability to focus tends to enhance the effect of the desensitization process, as the patient is exposed to the feared object or situation.[99]

Exposure to the feared situation or object may be achieved in a number of ways, including *direct actual exposure* to the feared entity (such as putting a person with fear of flying in a real airplane), *virtual reality exposure* (such as using computer or other simulations of the feared situation), or exposure through *guided imagery and visualization* (such as encouraging the person to imagine what it would be like to encounter the feared entity). A number of recent studies on a variety of different phobias, from fear of flying to fear of snakes, support these conclusions.

In a 2006 study,[100] University of Pennsylvania researchers found that patients with snake phobia could reduce their fears with mental imagery that had been modified by cognitive restructuring. Their fears were conveyed to them as mental suggestions in a rational context and were presented less starkly than would have been the case if they had confronted real snakes.

Another group of studies has established that mind body techniques can help with "blood phobias," which may be experienced by patients suffering traumatic injuries or donating blood. Just seeing blood may induce high anxiety, dizziness, nausea, or fainting. These studies have demonstrated the efficacy of mentally distracting techniques, such as relaxation exercises or "applied tension" of the muscles, a procedure that involves putting pressure on muscles in a part of the body that is separate from that part with the wound.

In one of these studies,[101] 30 patients with fear of blood coming from wounds and injuries were treated individually with applied tension, applied relaxation, or the combination of these two methods for a series of up to 10 sessions. They were assessed on self-reported, behavioral, and physiological measures before and after treatment and at a six-month follow-up. All groups improved significantly in overcoming their phobias according to 11 of 12 measurements, and they maintained their improvements at a six-month follow-up evaluation. The study showed that 73 percent of the patients had improved clinically at the end of the treatments and 77 percent had improved at a six-month follow-up.

In another study by a Canadian team, published in 2007 in *Transfusion*,[102] the researchers explored the use of mind body approaches to treat blood phobia symptoms associated with donation of blood. The phobic symptoms, they noted, may include dizziness, nausea, and fainting. Specifically, they evaluated the muscle-tensing technique of applied tension. In this context, applied tension referred to arranging for subjects to sit and assume postural positions that tense muscles in different parts of the body while the blood was being drawn. The researchers found that tension in the lower body was especially useful in reducing phobic symptoms and causing donors to agree to give blood again in the future.

A review article published in 2007 in *Clinical Psychology Review*[103] confirmed that a variety of lifestyle or mind body treatments work well in treating phobias. These treatments include in vivo (real-life) exposure to the feared object; virtual reality exposure; cognitive therapy; and "other treatments," which include relaxation therapy.

These techniques have been shown to help the problem for at least one year, according to the authors. Also, our own experience at the Benson-Henry Institute suggests that the symptoms associated with phobias can be controlled effectively in many people who employ a long-term version of our two-phase Benson-Henry Protocol.

The researchers concluded that most phobias respond "robustly" to real-life exposure. But this approach is associated with high dropout rates and low levels of acceptance of treatment—most likely because the patients find actual, unmitigated exposure to the feared entity too emotionally distasteful or overwhelming. "Systematic desensitization"—incremental or gradual exposure to the feared object or situation over time—appears to be more acceptable to most patients, though the authors noted that this approach has a more moderate success rate.

The investigators also reported that virtual reality exposure may be an effective treatment for fear of flying and fear of heights, but more controlled trials are needed to support this conclusion. They found that cognitive therapy—which we have sometimes coupled with Phase Two visualization—was most helpful in claustrophobia. This approach may involve changing the patient's mindset about a particular phobia through mental imagery.

For example, after going through the Phase One relaxation response trigger, the individual with claustrophobia might move into Phase Two by visualizing herself in a very small, tight elevator. The same exercise would be repeated daily for a week or two to achieve the desired desensitization and alleviation of the phobia.

Finally, the authors of this review on phobias confirmed the above findings about blood-injury phobia: This blood fear, they said, was uniquely responsive to applied tension, or tensing unrelated muscle groups as a distraction from the blood response.

Possible Mind Body Treatments

In applying an effective mind body treatment to counter certain problems with phobias, you should proceed through our two-phase protocol described on page 111.

A Case Study in Claustrophobia

Our two-phase treatment protocol worked particularly well in helping Jennifer overcome the claustrophobia that she typically experienced during certain diagnostic medical procedures. She especially had trouble when she was asked to enter a narrow, tube-shaped nuclear image scanning device that created computerized pictures of her heart. The medical procedure required her first to undergo a stress test on a treadmill. Then, during the last 30 seconds, she received an injection of a radioactive dye that was necessary for the production of the computerized images.

The problem was that the first time Jennifer was placed in the scanning tube, she experienced a classic claustrophobic attack, with rapid heart rate, shortness of breath, and an increasing sense of panic.

"I have to get out of here!" she told the technician, who immediately activated the platform on which she was lying and slid her out of the enclosed space.

Jennifer, the technician, and her cardiologist, who had been called in to the room, were in a quandary. She had successfully undergone her stress test, and time had been set aside for the scan. But the full diagnosis couldn't be completed unless she could somehow reenter the tube and submit to the scan, which she had been told would take about 12 to 15 minutes to complete.

"I've got a nice music tape I can play while you're in there," the technician said. "The sounds will help you go to a different place in your mind."

His words struck home with Jennifer because, luckily, she had been trained in our two-phase Benson-Henry Protocol for mind body healing. Before this incident, however, she had never connected her claustrophobia to the protocol she had learned and practiced. Her main focus, instead, had been on treating her mild hypertension, which had been largely cured by use of our protocol.

"Okay, I'll try it again," she said. "But I hope I'll like that music you're going to pipe in."

As it happened, the music was a sequence of Strauss's waltzes, which Jennifer had always found relaxing. But after she was ensconced in the tube and the scanner had moved down very close to her chest, she began to feel the claustrophobic panic again. The music obviously wasn't going to be enough to hold her attention and distract her from the scanning device, which increasingly seemed to be pinning her to the padded platform.

But she was determined to find a way out of her dilemma. She found herself thinking, "I know something about this mind body business— and I know it should work in this situation. So how about it?"

With this increased determination—and the music helping somewhat in the background—she began to move into a mind body approach that combined both phases of our protocol. A history buff, she had recently memorized all of the presidents of the United States in order. So she elected to move through a contemplation of each of them. As she named a particular president silently, she would allow her mind to drift into some event or achievement involving the man, and she would dwell on those thoughts for a short time. Then she would move on to the next president.

She first thought of Washington and recalled the painting that depicted him crossing the Delaware during the Revolutionary War. She imagined herself on the boat, rocking back and forth with the shivering American soldiers. Then she moved on to John Adams and saw him enjoying himself before a fire at his home in Braintree, Massachusetts, with his wife, Abigail. Jefferson was next. His name conjured up images of the signing of the Declaration of Independence.

She continued in this fashion through Madison, Monroe, John Quincy Adams, and Jackson—but then her reverie was interrupted.

"Okay, that does it," the technician's voice said from somewhere.

"It's been twelve minutes?" Jennifer asked as the platform moved out from the tube.

"Closer to fifteen," he said. "Nice job. You were really still during the entire procedure. Great pictures!"

Then Jennifer learned the bad news: She had to come back for a repeat procedure the following week so that the physicians would have comparative pictures of her heart at rest. At that point, she called me, saying, "I really don't think I can go through this again."

I reassured her that given the research that has been done on using mind body treatments for phobia, she could assume that her phobia was cured. She would be relaxed and in control during the next procedure. But to solidify her gains in overcoming this condition, I suggested that she use a form of desensitizing visualization daily for the next week preceding her second appointment. Each day she employed the Phase One relaxation response trigger and, immediately afterward, a Phase Two visualization in which she saw herself in the scanning tube.

At first, these desensitizing visualizations were somewhat disturbing: She could actually feel her breath growing shorter and anxiety creeping into her mind as she saw the scanner moving closer and closer to her body. But the symptoms were mild, and after a couple of days they disappeared. In the last few days of employing this type of desensitizing mental imagery, she actually began to enjoy herself.

When the time came for her second scan, Jennifer found herself looking forward to the experience, "just to see how well I can get through it." The insertion of her body into the tube and the restriction of her chest by the scanners were now familiar, and she sensed only a second or two of discomfort. Then, she was off on a journey in her mind, thinking of U.S. presidents and imagining major events in their lives.

Then the unexpected occurred. She sensed that the scanner had stopped, and the taped music had also ceased. But the technician had not pulled her out of the tube. In fact, she could hear him in the hallway talking to someone, apparently another patient whom he was preparing for the next scan.

"He's forgotten me," Jennifer thought.

She hadn't planned on this contingency, and the delay in releasing her from the scanner triggered a fear that grips many with claustrophobia: They worry that when they are confined in a close space, they will be there indefinitely, perhaps forever! Some anxiety and shortness of breath returned, but Jennifer concentrated on breathing regularly and went back to her presidents. When the technician walked back into the examining room and pulled her out of the tube, she was as calm as she had been before the procedure had begun. Clearly, her mind body approach to treatment had enabled her to make significant headway with her claustrophobia.

Premature Aging

Symptoms

The symptoms and signs of aging are all too familiar: wrinkled skin; deterioration of hearing, taste, and eyesight; decline in function of the reproductive system; loss of bone and muscle mass; reduced mental functioning; and the appearance of inherited diseases. The list goes on.

Of course, nothing can be done to eliminate aging or prevent death. There is no "cure" for growing old. But the onset of medical problems associated with advancing years may be slowed—and quality of life and physical function may be enhanced—through a number of measures available to all. These include regular medical examinations (and an appropriate patient's response to physicians' recommendations); proper use of various drugs and surgical procedures; and preventive medicine programs, which include regular aerobic exercise, improved nutrition, and stress-management techniques.

Standard Medical Treatments

A medical anti-aging sub-industry has grown in recent years. The offerings include plastic surgery, cataract and other eye surgery, and a variety of "drug cocktails" designed to ward off or minimize specific diseases.

Just as important, preventive medicine specialists have devised recommendations to slow the aging process. According to preventive medicine experts, the components of a preventive program that are most important in countering aging include 1) engaging in regular physical exercise, both aerobic and strength training; 2) reducing obesity; 3) not smoking; and 4) managing stress.[104] Again, this fourth preventive factor, the proper management of stress, falls mostly within the purview of mind body treatments.

Scientific Proof for Mind Body Approaches

Studies led by Sara Lazar of the Massachusetts General Hospital have employed functional magnetic resonance imaging (fMRI) technology. These investigations show that long-term meditation practice is associated with changes in the physical structure of the brain.[105] In a paper published in 2005 in *NeuroReport*, we evaluated 20 individuals with extensive experience in a type of meditation that required the participant to focus attention on internal experiences.

We found that the meditators' brain regions were thicker than average in the prefrontal cortex and right anterior insula (part of the right hemisphere of the brain). These parts of the brain are associated with attention, interoception (influencing organs in the viscera, such as the heart, liver, and intestines), and sensory processing. The increased cortical thickness was most pronounced in older participants, a fact that, in our opinion, suggested that meditation might offset age-related cortical thinning by slowing the rate of neural degeneration in certain parts of the brain.

Our findings provided the first structural evidence for "experience-dependent cortical plasticity" (ability of the brain to change) through the practice of the Phase One relaxation response. We suggested in our report that the parts of the brain affected by this meditation (the prefrontal cortex and right anterior insula) play a crucial role in adaptive decision making, cognitive functioning, and emotional processing.

In another Benson-Henry Institute study, published in 2006, we explored the use of the relaxation response as a mind body intervention to counteract the harmful effects of stress in aging adults.[106] Fifteen subjects were divided into two groups. The experimental group was given five successive weeks of relaxation response training; the second group, the control group, received no training. The average age of the participants was 71.3 years. At the end of the study, we found that the relaxation response–trained group achieved significant improvement on a simple task requiring basic mental and motor skills.

More research needs to be done into the impact of mind body treatments on memory and other mental functions among an aging population. Our research into the impact of the relaxation response on genetic activity associated with aging suggests that the mind body approach may be powerful in influencing the aging process.[107] We know enough now to recommend our two-phase mind body protocol to aging patients, both as a stress-reducer and also as a possible tool to enhance mental functioning.

Possible Mind Body Treatments

In applying an effective mind body treatment to help counter certain problems with premature aging, follow the basic two-phase Benson-Henry Protocol summarized on page 111.

Because "premature aging" is an amorphous term—and because the concept often overlaps with a variety of medical conditions related only tangentially to aging—you don't need to focus on a specific aspect of aging as you practice the basic protocol. The important thing is to delve into your memories and see yourself behaving vigorously and actively during Phase Two visualization.

So after you evoke the relaxation response in Phase One, you might "go back in time" in your mind and find a scene when you were youthful and active, a time when you sensed a great physical freedom. Perhaps you were playing on an athletic field, hiking vigorously, or taking a long, leisurely swim. Dwell on those moments for the 8 to 10 minutes of Phase Two. Savor the experience. Capture those times when you were particularly joyous and energetic in an outdoor setting.

After you have enjoyed this "remembered wellness" over a number of consecutive days and weeks, you may be pleasantly surprised to find that the *mental* experience begins to carry over into your *actual* daily life. You begin to feel more energetic—indeed, younger—as you go about ordinary tasks. If you allow yourself to believe that you are weak, downtrodden, unfortunate, and generally unhealthy, you're likely to feel the same negative way about your day-to-day experiences. You want to develop a mind that *heals,* rather than a mind that *injures.*

The Mind That Injures

We have written elsewhere about the "nocebo effect," the polar opposite of the placebo effect.[108] Too often, this mindset becomes fixed in aging patients, whose aspirations narrow as physical problems increase.

I'm reminded of one 93-year-old woman in a nursing facility who could be quite lucid and upbeat when she focused on lively discussions with visiting friends and relatives. But when she began to dwell on her more limited physical capacities—she needed to walk using a walker rather than under her own power—she became morose.

When she was in a "down" mood, one of her grown children reminded her that she would be executing a revised will that afternoon. Her mind enmeshed in negativity as she pondered this estate-planning task, she asked, "Am I dying? Is there something you're not telling me? Do I have a terminal illness?"

With such a depressed attitude, her energy level noticeably declined—until her son reminded her that every responsible person has to update a will now and then. In effect, he was encouraging her to visualize the positive side of this estate-preparation task. The suggestion took hold, and before long, she was feeling more energetic.

On a similar note, I have a patient who, in his mid-50s, suddenly developed hypertension. Upon questioning him, I learned that he had just reached the age when his father had died a premature death from causes related to cardiovascular problems, including high blood pressure. This man admitted that he had begun to fixate on his own blood pressure, a mental preoccupation that had obviously led to higher readings.

To help him counter this health problem, I taught him how to evoke the Phase One relaxation response. As it turned out, he didn't need any special instruction in visualization—that experience came automatically during Phase One. As he repeated his chosen focus phrase, he sensed he was in a zero-gravity environment, floating here and there like a human balloon. Within a couple of weeks, his blood pressure problem disappeared, along with worries that he was destined to follow his father to a premature death.

Premature Ventricular Contractions (Extra or Skipped Heartbeats) and Palpitations (Pounding Heartbeats)

Symptoms

Most people experience irregular heartbeats or a pounding heartbeat on occasion, and in most cases there is nothing to worry about. But some types of irregular or unusual heartbeats present more reasons for concern, especially when they occur frequently or are accompanied by other signs or symptoms, such as a fainting incident.

How can you tell if you are experiencing extra or skipped heartbeats?

One sign may be a pounding heartbeat (palpitation), which you can clearly feel for a short period in the center of your chest or upper abdomen. Palpitations occur because the heart "hesitates" before beating, causing a buildup of blood in one of the ventricles, the lower chambers of the heart. In releasing the extra blood, the heart pounds more intensely than normal, perhaps with an extra, quick beat. This type of skipping or extra-beat heart action is known as a premature ventricular contraction, or PVC.

You can also check for skipped or extra beats by taking your pulse: Gently press your fingers against the artery at the inside of the wrist. If the heartbeat you feel is irregular, you are experiencing skipped heartbeats, which could be PVCs. A variation on this phenomenon may include a sequence of very fast heartbeats (tachychardia) after slow beats. Or PVCs may occur with a very slow heart rate, perhaps slower than 40 beats per minute. If other symptoms, such as fainting, begin to occur with this condition, your physician will almost certainly refer you to a cardiologist for further evaluation.

A Note on Normal Heart Rates
The average resting heart rate range is 60 to 90 beats per minute, with normal resting rates sometimes rising to 100 beats per minute. Those with a resting rate below 60 beats per minute may be quite normal, but they are typically diagnosed as having bradycardia, a condition characterized by a heart rate lower than 60 beats per minute. This condition may be inherited or developed through prolonged endurance exercise training.

Standard Medical Diagnoses and Treatments
The cause for the type of heart rate irregularity known as PVCs may be the caffeine in the coffee you had this morning or a medication you're taking. Or the source of the problem may be aging or a congenital condition you inherited at birth. The best treatment for PVCs or skipped heartbeats may be simply to eliminate an offending food, drink, or medication.

One patient we know greatly reduced his PVCs and heart-pounding palpitations by reducing his intake of morning coffee from a prodigious five cups to one. Furthermore, he took this dietary step *after* consulting with his physician. If you determine that your heart is beating irregularly, is pounding, or is otherwise operating abnormally, make an appointment with your physician to be sure the cause of the problem is properly identified.

Your doctor may determine that your condition requires no further treatment, just regular medical monitoring. On the other hand, you may be a candidate for further evaluation and diagnosis by a cardiologist, who may order a stress test, an echocardiogram, or special procedures such as use of a Holter monitor (a device attached to your chest that records your heart behavior over a 24- to 48-hour period).[109]

Other times, a physical problem may be the culprit for PVCs. One example is "sick sinus syndrome," or a tendency of the heart's natural electrical systems to fail to send signals that "it's time for a beat." Such a diagnosis may require a medical intervention, such as the implantation of a pacemaker, to enable the heart to beat properly.

Scientific Proof for Mind Body Approaches

Our 2009 study on symptom management at the Benson-Henry Institute has identified frequent heart palpitations as one of the leading symptoms that responds well to mind body interventions.[110] (You'll recall that palpitations involve pounding heartbeats that may be accompanied by regular or irregular heartbeats.)

As for extra or skipped heartbeats (PVCs), we described in Chapter 4 on page 66 a 1975 *Lancet* study that I conducted with Sidney Alexander and Charles Feldman of the Harvard Medical School.[111] This investigation, which evaluated the effect of a regular elicitation of the relaxation response on PVCs, found that eight of 11 heart-disease patients experienced a reduced frequency of PVCs as a result of eliciting the relaxation response for 10 to 20 minutes twice daily for four weeks in their own homes, without medical supervision.

Later studies into related health conditions have confirmed this *Lancet* study. In a 1990 study published in *Behavioral Medicine,* I joined a Harvard Medical School team led by C. J. Hellman[112] to explore the effect of behavioral training and the relaxation response on a variety of symptoms with a "psychosocial component," including heart palpitations. We found that at the scheduled six-month follow-up, patients in the behavioral medicine groups showed significantly greater reductions in visits to physicians and also greater relief from discomforts involving physical and psychological symptoms than did the patients in the control group.

Other studies continue to reinforce these findings. Consider, for example, a 1996 study conducted at the University of Southern California Department of Nursing. The researchers found that, with a wide variety of stress symptoms including heart palpitations, "combination treatments"—drugs *plus* mind body interventions, such as relaxation therapy and cognitive coping strategies—have "high success rates."[113]

Possible Mind Body Treatments

An effective mind body treatment to counter irregular, extra, or skipped heartbeats and palpitations should include the two-phase protocol described on page 111.

A successful case history in which I was involved provides a useful model to show how our two-phase treatment protocol can work with a patient experiencing PVCs, or irregular heartbeats, with palpitations. The patient, Keith, in his mid-60s, had been experiencing extra or skipped heartbeats each day. Symptoms included a sense of tightness in the center of the chest and sometimes a pounding (palpitation) of the heart in the same location, especially at times of stress.

Because previous medical examinations, including resting and stress ECGs, had identified this condition years earlier, Keith had learned to check his pulse when he felt the sensations in his chest. In this way he could self-monitor how his heart rate correlated with his physical symptoms. He consistently found that his pulse hesitated or beat irregularly when the sensations occurred.

Also, Keith had been diagnosed when he was in his late 20s with bradycardia, or a naturally slow heart rate. Even when he was alert and pursuing daily activities, his resting heart rate would typically range from 50 to 55 beats per minute (remember, any heart rate below 60 is regarded as bradycardia). At night just before bedtime—or at other times of the day when he was particularly relaxed—his resting rate would go down into the low 40s and sometimes into the high 30s. From what his physicians had been able to ascertain, Keith had apparently had this benign condition all his life, with rates in the lowest ranges occurring when he was in particular good physical and aerobic shape.

These symptoms had no impact on Keith's ability to function until he suffered a fainting incident after urinating early one morning. While he was standing at the lavatory, he felt lightheaded and then found himself sitting on the bathroom floor. The incident seemed to have lasted only a second or two, and he suffered no injuries. But he was concerned enough to bring up the matter with his primary physician, an internist.

This doctor placed Keith on a Holter monitor, which was strapped to his chest and recorded his heart rate and electrical activity for 24 hours. The results showed that on occasion Keith's heart rate went much lower than he had expected, with the lowest rate occurring briefly at just under 30 beats per minute. This primary care physician tentatively diagnosed Keith with sick sinus syndrome,[114] characterized by a failure of the heart to receive proper electrical signals to stimulate heartbeats.

"What happens if I don't do anything about this?" Keith asked.

"You could faint again and hurt yourself this time," said the doctor, who routinely talked freely with his patients. "Or the delays in the heartbeats could increase in length or frequency."

"And what if the delays last a long time?"

"You could have a stroke or die." But he noted that this danger was very improbable.

Keith appreciated his doctor's forthrightness, and he also got the point.

"So what's the next step?" he asked.

"You have to see a cardiologist for further tests—and you may need a demand pacemaker," the doctor told Keith, referring to the common electronic device implanted in the chest, which sends electrical signals to the heart when the heart rate slows down too much (most of the time, the heart continues to beat on its own without this device being activated).

So the physician referred Keith to a cardiologist for a final decision. But as Keith was waiting for the appointment with the heart specialist, he found himself worrying that he might have another fainting incident, which could result in injury. Also, his PVCs and palpitations seemed to be occurring more often.

At this point, I entered the picture and began to advise him about the use of mind body treatments to supplement the evaluations and recommendations he was getting from his other physicians. I pointed out that the fears he was feeling about falling again and also the increased number of PVCs and palpitations might well have been the result of increased stress and anxiety. Also, I said, the stress component would respond well to a mind body strategy.

"This is the right time to begin to employ a mind body approach," I said.

Keith then chose to follow our two-phase Benson-Henry Protocol. He employed the Phase One relaxation response trigger at least once a day for 12 to 15 minutes the first thing in the morning. Sometimes he would repeat the exercise later in the day—a perfectly acceptable variation on the basic protocol. His focus of attention for Phase One varied from centering on his breathing, to watching the lights and shapes floating behind his eyelids, to repetitive prayers. Also, throughout the day he consistently used a "mini" Phase One procedure by employing his focus of attention for short periods, sometimes no longer than 15 seconds. (See the earlier description in this chapter, page 116.)

Keith also utilized Phase Two visualization for 8 to 10 minutes after each regular, full-length Phase One session. During these imagery experiences, he constructed a mental picture of himself moving about and doing his daily tasks in various settings. Whenever he saw himself going into the bathroom, he visualized a state of good health, emotional assurance, and confidence. Another way of describing Keith's Phase Two is that he remembered—and, in a mental sense, began to "live in"—healthy states he had enjoyed in the past, with absolutely no fear of fainting.

Sometimes in his mental "pictures" he would recall the fainting incident, and that could trigger a brief sense of apprehension or fear. But after we discussed these experiences, he learned to expect those intrusive images and to turn away from them each time with an "Oh well." The negative memories of the fainting may even have been useful as a mind body treatment, because they began to serve as a desensitizing factor. As he exposed himself mentally to the fear of fainting, he became desensitized to the fear and actually became less afraid of that possibility.

After two weeks Keith found that his fears of fainting had subsided, and he also experienced fewer PVCs and palpitations. Then he went in for his appointment with the cardiologist. After undergoing a battery of tests, Keith was informed that his condition was not serious and that unless he had other symptoms, he would not need a pacemaker.

"You're in good shape," the cardiologist said.

The wave of relief that came with this news, along with the positive impact of the two-phase mind body protocol, caused Keith to put the fainting episode out of his mind. Now, when he goes into the bathroom early in the mornings, he never fears a fainting incident.

So what happened inside Keith to bring about this change?

First, the two-phase Benson-Henry Protocol he had employed for more than three months achieved the physiologic effect that our research says it can achieve: The frequency of extra or skipped heartbeats decreased significantly, and the heart-pounding incidents, or palpitations, were reduced.

Second, the various physiologic changes that occur with the relaxation response came into play, including lowered blood pressure, a calmer and slower rate of breathing, control of hormones and neurotransmitters associated with stress, and a calming of the mind, with less anxiety.

Third, we can assume from our genetic research that Keith's daily elicitations of the relaxation response over a period in excess of eight weeks—or the training period we used for our experimental groups—had begun to change his gene activity or expression. The "package" of genes associated with anti-stress responses had been "switched on" by Keith's practice of the two-phase mind body protocol. As a result, his body and emotions were now operating in a way that protected him from the PVCs, palpitations, and various fears that had helped trigger the physiologic responses.

Premenstrual Syndrome (PMS)

Symptoms

Premenstrual syndrome (PMS), a medical condition that arises between a woman's ovulation and menstruation when the ovaries produce progesterone, troubles an estimated 75 percent of ovulating women.

Symptoms may include irritability, depression, mood swings, problems with concentration or memory, physical fatigue, a craving for salty or sweet foods, abdominal bloating and pain, swollen hands or feet, tender breasts, and nausea or other gastrointestinal upsets.[115]

Standard Medical Treatments

In treating PMS symptoms, medical experts typically recommend lifestyle changes, such as dietary adjustments and increased exercise, before they prescribe medications.[116] Common lifestyle remedies include changes in diet, such as taking more calcium (1,200 milligrams per day), magnesium, vitamin B_6, and vitamin E. Also, many medical experts urge avoiding nicotine, caffeine, alcohol, and salt. Increasing aerobic exercise may also help relieve PMS symptoms by promoting feelings of well-being after a workout.

More aggressive standard medical treatments involve the prescribing of drugs such as antidepressant serotonin reuptake inhibitors and pain receptor inhibitors. Other, more extreme possibilities are drugs that can limit or block the production of estrogen, but these can have serious side effects, such as causing symptoms of menopause and increasing the risk of bone loss through osteoporosis.[117]

Because stress is often a factor in PMS, a preferable approach—in addition to the dietary and exercise options—is stress-reduction techniques. As mentioned in Chapter 4 on page 68, Nancy Rigotti, of the Massachusetts General Hospital and the Harvard Medical School, writing in the *Harvard Medical School Family Health Guide,* has recommended "practicing stress reduction techniques" for PMS, "such as the relaxation response."[118]

Scientific Proof for Mind Body Approaches

In a 1990 report in *Obstetrics & Gynecology,* Irene Goodale, Alice Domar, and I—all from Harvard Medical School and New England Deaconess Hospital—explored the use of mind body treatments to relieve PMS symptoms. The study, which we cited on page 68, involved 46 women who were suffering from PMS. We found that those with the most severe symptoms showed significant improvement after eliciting the relaxation response for five months. Our conclusion: regular elicitation of the relaxation response was an effective treatment for the physical and emotional symptoms of PMS, and was "most effective in women with severe symptoms."[119]

Our findings have been confirmed in a variety of later investigations. For example, scientists from the Department of Psychiatry, University of Connecticut Medical School, conducted a review in 2006 on the effects of meditation techniques on various types of illness.[120] Among other things, they determined that the strongest evidence for the medical efficacy of meditative techniques could be found in treatments for PMS and menopause.

A team of French researchers reported in 2001 that training in relaxation techniques "is particularly suitable" for treatment of PMS symptoms.[121] Other studies that have found relaxation therapy to be useful include a 2003 report in *Psychoneuroendocrinology*[122] and various investigations of specific meditative techniques, such as specialized yoga exercises.[123]

Possible Mind Body Treatments

An effective mind body treatment to counter the symptoms of PMS should begin with the two-phase Benson-Henry Protocol summarized on page 111.

If you have PMS symptoms, we recommend that you incorporate the above two-phase protocol into your daily personal health plan. The cited studies show that the elicitation of the relaxation response in Phase One is an absolutely essential part of the mind body treatment. In addition, our research into how the relaxation response influences gene expression provides strong evidence that any stress-related causes of your symptoms may be alleviated throughout your gene activity.

Also, Phase Two will prove helpful in reinforcing the Phase One experience and in bolstering your expectation-belief that the research findings we have cited not only work for others but also possess the power to work for you. Here is a suggestion for the type of visualization you might use:

Spend a few minutes recalling situations where PMS symptoms have interfered with your normal activities. Perhaps you have felt that you couldn't engage in sports or family activities when you were experiencing abdominal pains or other PMS discomforts.

Now, picture in your mind those same activities at other times of the month—or when you have been able to enjoy the events without discomfort, pain, or excessive fatigue. Hold those enjoyable memories or images in your mind for the full 8 to 10 minutes of each visualization session. See the scenes from multiple perspectives and at different times. As you observe these activities mentally, continue to breathe at a normal, rhythmic rate. When thoughts of your PMS discomfort break into your train of thought—and they *will* break in, you can be sure of that—just smile to yourself, turn away from them, and return to your pleasant memory.

As you engage in these mind body treatments for PMS symptoms, always remember that the best, proven remedies for the discomforts you are feeling lie in the mind body realm. You really can relieve your problems with this condition if you commit yourself to developing an expertise as a "mind body practitioner"—a goal that is entirely within your grasp if you just follow the recommendations we are making here.

And These Treatments Are Just the Beginning . . .

The above mind body guide for treating numerous medical conditions is by no means intended to represent an exhaustive list. On the contrary, these treatments are just the beginning. The possibilities for applying mind body approaches will expand in the years ahead as new research is performed on specific diseases. In the meantime, whatever medical condition you confront, you can be confident that the two-phase protocol we are describing in these pages will be useful, either by itself or as an adjunct to other standard medical procedures. The treatment potential of the two-phase mind body protocol increases with those medical conditions that have a significant stress component.

Diseases in which our two-phase mind body approach should be useful are those in which the placebo effect has been shown to be effective.[124] These include, but are not limited to, the following:

- Allergic skin reactions
- Bronchial asthma
- Congestive heart failure
- Constipation
- Cough
- Diabetes mellitus
- Drowsiness
- Duodenal ulcers
- Fatigue and dizziness
- Herpes simplex (cold sores)
- Hostility and anger, which have been linked to heart attacks

- Impotency, related to stress or performance anxiety
- Obesity
- Postoperative swelling
- Post-traumatic stress disorder (PTSD)
- Tinnitus, or sensation of sounds

These conditions represent a few in the growing list of medical problems that respond to mind body treatments, according to preliminary research and clinical experience. But they are only the beginning of the story. Our ongoing genetic research is revealing still other possibilities for treatment—possibilities that hold promise for countering some of the most serious diseases we face.

8.

Cancer and the Genetic Horizons of Mind Body Treatment

ameron, 32 years old but already a wealthy and successful investor, contacted me from another part of the country to say that he was suffering from a rare type of leukemia. Cameron was just exceeding the estimated two-year time limit he had been given to live. He had undergone chemotherapy and other standard treatments, but he said he wanted to leave no option untried. He was particularly concerned about the impact that his death might have on his wife and child. So he was wondering what relaxation response approaches I might suggest for him to investigate in the area of mind body treatment.

During our discussion, he noted that he was experiencing intermittent scaling and itching of the skin (pruritus), reactions that may be associated with chemotherapy or a combination of chemotherapy and radiation. Also, he had encountered occasional bouts with nausea and vomiting from the chemotherapy.

"So is there any mind body approach that might help me?" he asked.

I responded that I could not establish a physician-patient relationship with him over the phone or offer him any formal medical treatment in that way. But I said that I could introduce him to our generic mind body approach to healing—our two-phase protocol. Then, he could share the information with his physician and, under his doctor's supervision, begin to employ some of the mind body techniques that I would describe.

To reinforce his acceptance and belief in what I was suggesting, and also his expectation that the mind body approach could be of use to him, I noted what you already know from reading this book: Scientific studies have established that our Phase One relaxation response training and other mind body techniques, such as desensitization, can relieve nausea, vomiting, and other symptoms related to chemotherapy.[1] I thought this information would be important for him since there was a chance he might require chemotherapy again.

Also, as indicated above, pruritus, which is sometimes accompanied by scaling of the skin, may result from chemotherapy *or* from certain forms of cancer, including different types of leukemia.[2] The good news for leukemia patients like Cameron is that a body of scientific evidence is emerging that relaxation "stress training" and "relaxation techniques," among other mind body approaches, are important elements in the treatment of scaling and pruritus.[3]

Finally, I knew that our new genetic research showed that eliciting the relaxation response for at least eight weeks could influence his gene activity so as to trigger gene expressions that would be the opposite of those associated with stress. If stress was a factor in his illness, our approach might be of use. At that point, even I did not quite grasp the full implications of this genetic point—as you will see as Cameron's story unfolds.

Because he was interested in taking some practical steps that might help him, I described over the phone a version of our two-phase protocol. But to keep things simple, I suggested that he might want to begin only with Phase One, the evocation of the relaxation response. So I described the basic eight-step procedure summarized in the box in Chapter 7 on page 111.

I was particularly cautious with Cameron because I was keenly aware of how some author-physicians who promote certain ideas about healing or treatment may go too far. They may enthusiastically promise a miraculous cure from some diet, dietary supplement, lifestyle adjustment, mental program, or spiritual panacea—even though such approaches are unsupported by scientific research or consistent clinical experience. The end result of such unfounded enthusiasm is, more often than not, a failure of the "miraculous" treatment to heal and an overwhelming sense of guilt, disappointment, failure, or blame, both in the patient and in loved ones who may have suggested trying the unproven approach.

Despite my caution, I felt comfortable demonstrating Phase One because, given all the science support, I was confident the self-treatment would stand a good chance of counteracting harmful stress. In any case, the protocol couldn't hurt and was safe.

After our phone call, Cameron's case receded to the back of my mind—until our genetic research generated another dramatic finding: We established a link between the relaxation response and genetic activity that has been associated with various cancers, including leukemia.

The Cancer Connection

You will recall that in our initial genetic research, we determined that gene activity caused by the relaxation response (Phase One of our treatment protocol) directly counters or opposes gene activity induced by stress.[4] In the research that came to light shortly after my telephone conversation with Cameron, we examined whether the gene expression or activity triggered by the relaxation response could also be associated with gene expression associated with different types of cancers.[5]

To perform this research, our Institute team used results from the same two groups who had participated in our original research. One group included short-term relaxation response trainees, who had undergone eight weeks of mind body training. The other group was composed of long-term practitioners of the relaxation response, who had employed mind body techniques for an average of more than nine years. But for this cancer study, we employed a somewhat different methodology.

The distinguishing feature of this new study, with Manoj Bhasin as first author, was that we compared our findings involving our relaxation response practitioners with cancer databases compiled by the Broad Institute of Massachusetts Institute of Technology and Harvard, and the Weizmann Institute of Science in Israel. These databases identify cancer gene "signatures" or "sets," which are associated with groups of gene activity of different cancer patients. Specifically, we determined whether gene sets in our relaxation response subjects might correlate with cancer-associated gene sets in cancer patients.

The results of our investigation were presented at the Society for Integrative Oncology, 6th International Conference, in 2009. The findings were rather startling and highly encouraging for future research and possible medical treatment. We found that the gene set expression in the long-term relaxation response practitioners in our study was *counter to* the gene expression in various cancers: lymphoma (follicular and B cell lymphoma), neuro tumors (central nervous system and glioma), liver, leukemia (myeloid, acute promyelocytic, B cell chronic leukemia), multiple myeloma, B cell chronic lymphoblastic leukemia, and another form of leukemia. Also, the results from these long-term practitioners showed gene set expression that was in the same direction as, or consistent with, the expression found in certain anticancer therapies.

As for the short-term trainees—who had started with no background in mind body techniques, but who had been instructed in and practiced our Phase One relaxation response approach for eight weeks—the results were also encouraging. Their relaxation response gene set expression signatures countered or opposed the gene signatures for such cancers as neuro tumors, multiple myeloma, and leukemia.

A Step Toward a Cancer Treatment Strategy

It was difficult for me *not* to see certain possible connections between Cameron's cancer and this new genetic research. After all, he was suffering from a leukemia, and our findings showed that the relaxation response could counter genetic activity associated with various leukemias.

However, I was cautious in advising him, as I would be with any other cancer patient. I had to stay strictly within the limits of our research findings. I especially had to be careful not to give false hope, even as I might interpret such findings to provide reasonable encouragement.

And there did seem to be some grounds for hope. With these new, significant cancer results, we found that the gene set activity in cancer patients ran in one direction, while the activity of the same group of genes in relaxation response (Phase One) practitioners ran in the opposite direction. For anyone in the healing profession who might be counseling a patient suffering from one of the cancers we had studied, that had to be an encouraging sign.

But at the same time, there were profound limits to what I might promise. For one thing, our relaxation response subjects were *all healthy—none suffered from cancer.* Because these original findings were "hypothesis-generating" and needed to be replicated, many additional rounds of research were absolutely necessary. Those future investigations would directly compare *only cancer patients* who employed or did not employ the Phase One relaxation response protocol.

I could not yet tell any cancer patients, including Cameron, "There is a new, established treatment for your cancer."

I *could* say, however, "There is new research that represents a promising first step toward a new cancer therapy. And, at the very least, this approach is safe and could make you feel better."

Serendipitously, Cameron had called me to say he wanted to coordinate a business trip to Boston so that he could see me and follow up on our initial phone conversation. When we met, he said that he had been practicing the Phase One elicitation of the relaxation response daily. As a result, he felt much less anxious, and his scaling and itching symptoms had lessened. As cited earlier, that improvement might have been linked to the impact of the relaxation response training on the leukemia itself. Because he had finished his chemotherapy months earlier, he felt, quite reasonably I thought, that improvement in his leukemia through the relaxation response might be the reason.

During our conversation, I mentioned in very general terms the encouraging leukemia findings in our research. At the same time, I cautioned him against expecting anything when our research was at such an early stage. But I felt that, as a leukemia patient, he was entirely justified in employing our Phase One approach because it continued to make him feel better, it was safe, and it just *might* help him. Furthermore, I felt that, as a physician, I would be acting irresponsibly if I knew a certain treatment could help a patient with a serious, even terminal illness but failed to use my advance knowledge about our research to do anything about it.

Cameron's Case: A Preliminary Cancer Treatment Model

In many ways, Cameron's case provides us with a model of how to pursue mind body treatments for cancer, even without final, definitive medical findings. Several guidelines derived from his situation may show the way:

- First, you should undergo routine treatment by an oncologist. If chemotherapy is involved, Phase One relaxation response therapy could counteract related nausea, vomiting, or other symptoms during this routine treatment.
- Second, the knowledge that you have cancer is stressful by itself, so symptoms you experience may be related to your knowledge

of, and worries about, the cancer. Our two-phase protocol could be of use here.

- Finally, a realistic understanding of what is known scientifically about mind body treatments for your particular condition—and also what is not known—is essential.

If you rely on wishful thinking or unsubstantiated rumor about different "alternative" medicine treatments, faddish cure-all diets, or unproven supplements, you may be sorely disappointed or even be hurt in the final results. Just as serious, you or your loved ones who have advocated an unsupported treatment may begin to experience remorse, anger, or guilt, perhaps because you feel you have wasted your time with ineffectual treatments, or even that your attempts to travel an unproven path have actually done harm.

But if you are aware of the scientific realities of mind body treatments, you will be much more likely to believe in them and achieve the best results. Anti-stress treatments, as well as genetically based approaches that are in the preliminary stages of research, can be used *at the same time* that you are getting the full benefits from standard treatments. Furthermore, the two-phase Benson-Henry Protocol won't expose you to harm.

Your ultimate objective in combining preliminary mind body cancer research and standard medical procedures should be to create a win-win scenario for yourself. Your goal should be twofold: With your doctor's guidance, maximize your use of the traditional, reductionistic medical system. At the same time, take advantage of safe—and possibly effective—mind body approaches to treatment, as good science points the way. Leave no therapeutic stone unturned—cover all responsible options.

As you move into the realm of mind body treatment for cancer and other disorders, you are likely to find yourself exploring horizons that cannot be completely explained or analyzed by reductionist, scientific research techniques. It is at this point that you enter an area of medical research and treatment that scientists have called "emergence," where the whole is greater than the sum of its parts.

Part III

The Possibilities of Mind Body Medicine

9.

The Whole Is Greater Than
the Sum of Its Parts

I have been at the Harvard Medical School as a student, trainee, and faculty member, respectively, for almost 50 years. Throughout my career, Harvard Medical School science has been, and still is, almost exclusively reductionistic. I was educated in and conducted my career in that model.

But what exactly do we mean when we talk about "reductionism"?

You'll recall that the term refers to the prevailing approach to modern scientific research that assumes all our understanding about the world can be reduced to the particular parts of any given topic or issue. According to this view of reality, to treat or cure cancer or diabetes we must first identify the causes of such diseases down to their molecular components. Only then can we work our way back up to a complete understanding of the disease. Those who affirm reductionism assume, in effect, that the whole is *equal to* the sum of its parts.

Certainly, reductionism has been absolutely necessary for us to reach our current, advanced stage of medical progress. Without reductionistic approaches in our research, scientists would never have achieved such medical breakthroughs as antibiotics and advanced surgical techniques. But reductionism can go only so far—as I have found out during my career.

My Uneasy Life as a Reductionist

As mentioned previously, using this scientifically approved, reductionistic methodology, I discovered the relaxation response in the same room at Harvard Medical School where the fight-or-flight response was discovered half a century before by Walter B. Cannon. But the relaxation response did not fully conform to reductionistic science. Certainly, the phenomenon involved a biological event that was associated with measurable, predictable, and reproducible physiologic and biochemical changes. My colleagues and I have utilized evolving reductionistic technologies, including those involving genetic research, to better understand the relaxation response. But there is a problem: The relaxation response is characterized by extremely complex mind body interactions that cannot be completely measured in reductionistic terms.

Because of this paradox, I found myself entangled in an academic trap: I was standing outside the medical establishment, grappling with reductionistic challenges at every turn, even as I was working within that same establishment.

On one level, Harvard Medical School, despite its reductionism, has proved to be a supportive environment to pursue my hard-to-define career in mind body medicine. In the early 1970s, for instance, I was awarded $300,000—in today's dollars, more than $1.5 million—from a private foundation to study an Eastern mind body technique, Transcendental Meditation. Yet some at the Medical School questioned whether or not I should be allowed to accept the monies to study such practices, which they regarded as far beyond the pale of accepted medical research. This project simply was not seen as sufficiently "scientific" (an objection that could be translated as "reductionistic").

To discuss my case, I secured a meeting with the dean of the Harvard Medical School, Robert Ebert. He concluded our discussion by stating, "If Harvard can't take a chance, who can? Take the money!"

After his retirement from the Medical School, Ebert demonstrated his support anew: He became the chairman of the board of directors of the Mind/Body Medical Institute, which I had founded with several colleagues in 1988. This Institute, which pursued research into a wide variety of mind body areas, was succeeded in 2006 by the Benson-Henry Institute for Mind Body Medicine at Massachusetts General Hospital.

But the Harvard Medical School environment was not always so supportive of new approaches. In the late 1970s, my chief of medicine, who was my boss and a noted reductionist, convened a review panel of non-Harvard academics to assess whether my research had an adequate scientific basis.

The final report of the panel was ambivalent, and my chief concluded that I would be allowed to continue my work at Harvard provided I conformed to two criteria within two years: First, I had to publish new findings in a highly respected scientific journal, whose criteria for acceptance observed the rules of vigorous reductionistic science; and second, I was required to obtain a National Institutes of Health competitive grant, which always involved reviewers who utilize highly reductionistic criteria. I fulfilled both criteria by publishing in *Science* and being awarded an NIH grant—and I was allowed to continue my work at Harvard Medical School. Now, after 30 years, Harvard Medical School is advocating "translational research," an approach based on cross-disciplinary linkages of the type that I have been pursuing since the beginning of my career.

Unrelenting Reductionistic Pressure

Because of ongoing academic pressure, my colleagues and I have been careful to insist on the use of standard, reductionistic, scientific methodology in our subsequent research to make the case for mind body approaches. In recommending mind body techniques, we have emphasized those treatments that are backed by such research protocols and tools as double-blind, controlled studies; random selection of subjects; functional magnetic resonance imaging (fMRI); and sophisticated genetic technology, such as microarray analysis (see Chapter 2, page 22).

Employing the reductionistic approach has been necessary to counter objections, made by proponents of reductionistic science, to mind body phenomena and treatments. We knew that reductionists would find it hard to oppose findings based on their own approach to research, even though those findings establish the validity and usefulness of the relaxation response, the placebo effect, and other mind body phenomena.

The Limits of Reductionism

Yet are these reductionistic criteria comprehensive enough to enable us to understand completely advanced reductionistic concepts such as genetics? The committed reductionist would argue that our very lives can be reduced to genetic interactions. For example, when the human genome sequencing was finished a few years ago, scientists expected that their knowledge could soon be used to treat every disease, especially cancer.[1]

But the world of genetics has proven to be much too complex for such reductionism. The basic hereditary configurations of genes, made up of DNA, are extraordinarily complicated, and their expression is continuously being modified within our bodies. There are countless subunits of DNA with gene expressions that are being modified second by second by second! Each of these modifications endlessly influences many others. Every moment of our lives, our bodies are different and changing. And new research findings frequently revise the rules that dictate these modifications. As the genetics story unfolds, reductionism is proving to be a woefully inadequate approach for analyzing this incredibly dynamic system of biology. In fact, biology in general has been called "irreducibly complex" by at least one expert.[2]

A similar kind of analysis can be applied to medical treatment. It is generally assumed, for instance, that most of the health problems in patients with diabetes are caused by elevated blood glucose levels. A logical conclusion, then, is that control of glucose levels should improve or cure the patient's condition. But according to a 2008 commentary by Henry H. Q. Heng in the *Journal of the American Medical Association,* controlling glucose levels actually increased the risks of death.[3]

Another illustration of this phenomenon, which was mentioned by Heng, involves chemotherapy.[4] Citing two cancer studies, he noted that chemotherapy may reduce the size of tumors at the outset of treatment. But then the treatment may produce other tumors, along with additional negative side effects.[5]

Many other examples of the failure of a limited medical response to solve a broad, systemwide medical problem also come to mind. Liposuction, which involves the surgical removal of fatty tissue deposits as a corrective for obesity or as a cosmetic measure to eliminate unsightly bulges, may at first seem a direct, appropriate remedy for the overweight. But this one-track method of getting rid of fat carries many risks for the patient and may have no impact on the underlying causes of the obesity, such as a patient's lack of motivation to eat a healthier, lower-calorie diet or to exercise. The end result may be a temporary loss of some fat but then a long-term gain of more weight.

Drugs that counter insomnia may work as a reductionistic treatment for a short period of time (see Chapter 7, page 135). But sleep medications rarely solve the problem over the long term and may lead to drug side effects, such as worsened quality of sleep or addiction, which leave the patient's health in an even worse state than its pre-drug condition.[6]

So what is the antidote to medical reductionism? An answer may lie in the mind body arena.

The Search for an Antidote to Reductionism

Mind body approaches to treatment suggest some interesting avenues to overcome the traps of reductionistic treatment. One promising possibility involves the broad, whole-body healing potential of mind body approaches, such as expectation-belief, the relaxation response, and various forms of cognitive therapy.

A certain mind body treatment may help hypertension, depression, or insomnia. At the same time, this treatment will counter the *overall* physical and mental manifestations of stress through the calming of brain activity and altering hormones and gene expression. The mind body treatment performs particular, reductionistic functions on specific health complaints *and at the same time* tends to the health of the *entire* biological system. The standard approaches to treatment, such as medications and surgery, do not perform such broad functions. Instead, their impact tends to be limited to particular symptoms and disorders.

So in the quest for a viable, practical mind body antidote to reductionistic limitations, the tools of reductionism must be temporarily abandoned and other tools must be found to enable us to understand the full significance of mind body treatments. With this goal in mind, let's now explore in a little more detail the meaning of that paradoxical statement that has introduced this chapter: "The whole is greater than the sum of its parts."

Why the Whole May Be Greater

This paradox—"the whole is greater than the sum of its parts"— may have profound implications for medical research and treatment, including your approach to your own health. But what exactly does it mean—and is it really valid?

A rather mundane way of understanding this principle may be found in athletics, politics, business management, or other fields involving intense competition. Most of us have become captivated by the unlikely competitor who, "on paper," just did not seem to have the ability or experience to vie for a top spot or championship. Analysts or oddsmakers tend to write off these Cinderella contestants, at least at first. But when the dark horse becomes a contender or a winner, onlookers become excited and fascinated. Somehow, the "parts" of long-shot competitors—the known expertise, training, and previous records—did not add up to the "whole" of their stellar performance. And pundits typically spend hours trying to figure out how the improbable outcome could have occurred.

Although many credit Aristotle with the "whole is greater" saying[7]—and it is true that some sections of his works suggest this principle—the concept has more recently been associated with certain theories associated with scientific research and medical treatment. The journal *Science* probed this issue in some depth in its July 2009 issue, with a particular focus on how physicists are recognizing that complex socioeconomic systems and networks have escaped the understanding of those who attempt to analyze only the workings of their component parts.

According to this argument, highly complicated systems such as traffic patterns, economic networks, and even human emotions simply cannot be defined by looking at the individual elements of each system. Instead, the *Science* report says, the interaction of these elements leads to "emergent behavior" that "makes the group more than the sum of its parts."[8]

The Whole Body in Medicine

In treating diabetes or other diseases, or in the socioeconomic realm, as the *Science* article demonstrates, the reductionistic approach may not work well. Yet reductionistic medical science continues to teach that the sum of basic research findings—that is, the discoveries about physiologic responses, molecular changes, or genetic activity of the human body—if modified, will correct the disorder. Still, in our research into mind body phenomena, a basic question has constantly nagged away: Can the whole totality *really* be fully understood by using such a reductionistic approach?

As Henry H. Q. Heng has argued in his 2008 article in the *Journal of the American Medical Association,* major medical problems can arise when a reductionist approach to treatment runs head-on into a complex biological system. He poses the issue this way:

"Most medical treatments make sense based on research of specific molecular pathways, so why do unexpected consequences occur after years of treatment? More simply, does the treatment that addresses a specific disease-related component harm the individual as a whole?"[9]

In answering his own questions, he concedes that many medical therapies—including antibiotics, pacemakers, blood transfusions, and organ transplants—have often succeeded, despite their reductionistic emphasis. They were designed to treat a particular problem or symptom related to a broader medical condition, and they have in fact worked as treatments.

But he cautions that when a system is "on the edge of chaos," employing a single response or a limited group of responses may actually pitch the entire system into a chaotic or harm-producing state. A human body on the verge of serious disease, for instance, may be pushed over the edge by just one additional drug or surgical procedure. He goes on to cite various responses to drug therapy, including harmful side effects, as signs that a particular therapy may have placed undue stress on the overall bodily functions.

What might be done to guard against these reductionistic problems in medical treatment?

Heng suggests that a gradual approach to certain treatments, rather than a "drastic intervention," may lead to a better result. But perhaps most important of all, we need to keep in mind that the *entire* body needs to be considered when we are treating one part of the body. If we can somehow care for the whole body at the same time that we focus on medical treatments for particular parts of the body, we may end up with a much better treatment result. The risks must continuously be weighed against the benefits.

But what exactly do we really know about the *whole* nature of our bodies and minds? And more to the point, how can we incorporate what we know into our personal treatment plans? To answer, we need to explore the phenomenon of *emergence.*

The Principle of Emergence

As indicated at the beginning of this chapter, our own interdisciplinary research at the Benson-Henry Institute is based on reductionistic methodologies. We have always been careful to observe all necessary reductionistic scientific protocols as we have studied how the relaxation response influences genetic expression; brain activity; molecular interactions, such as the release of nitric oxide; and other physiologic responses, such as blood pressure. But the more progress we make with our reductionistic research, including our work in the field of genetics, the more we realize what we are uncovering is so complex that we may never find a complete explanation.

To use terms that are gaining currency in medical research, there appear to be *emergent* or *synergistic* properties inherent in biological systems. Emergence in a philosophical medical context carries with it the implication that the whole of a human biological system is somehow greater than its constituent elements. Or to put this another way, the health and survival of the entire body often depend on more than just adjusting one or a few parts of the body.

A term that is related to emergence and is sometimes used synonymously with it is *synergism.* The common definition of synergism is the process by which separate, distinct parts of any system interact in such a way that the total effect of all the interactions is greater than the effect of any single interaction.

Examples of synergism may include the operation of an entire economy, as individual industries, agencies, and consumers interact in the real world. Another illustration that is sometimes offered is the total effect of drug interactions in the body, which may produce an overall dangerous or lethal effect even though the actions of an individual drug, given by itself, may be beneficial.

Now, in terms of your own health, how might you capture the positive forces of emergence or synergism as you deal with particular health conditions?

Capturing the Power of the Whole

The starting point for capturing the power of whole health in your life is to recognize that we know with considerable certainty at least three things about how reductionism and emergence (or synergism) may work together to enhance to your health:

First, emergent phenomena must be anchored in reductionistic proof. Without such an anchor, the validity of an emergent phenomenon would become a theory without documented, practical usefulness. The two must work together, bolstering each other. On a practical level, this means that before you consider any nontraditional medical claim, you should look closely to see whether that claim can be backed up in any way by standard, reductionistic research.

Second, despite the benefits, there are also definite limits to reductionistic medical research and treatment. If you rely only on reductionistic medicine for healing, you may find that your maximum healing potential is quite limited. Harm may even result from a given reductionistic treatment in the form of side effects of drugs, unexpected complications of surgery or other procedures, or other unintended results. So you must find a way to protect yourself against reductionistic excesses.

To achieve such protection, you should focus on working with your physician to integrate mind body techniques into your treatment program. Ask your doctor about the possibility of safely using fewer medications and surgeries. As you work together, you and your physician should regularly monitor the effect of any reductionistic treatment on your *whole* body.

Third, make use of the lessons and suggestions contained in this book. Throughout, we have tried to provide you with a comprehensive mind body approach to a variety of health problems; at the same time, we have shown you ways to balance mind body strategies and standard medical treatments. In fact, we have become convinced that the application of the mind body medical treatments described in Chapter 7 (page 109) is one of the best ways now available for any patient to achieve his or her maximum health potential.

But there is still more to this rather elusive concept of emergence. Experiences entirely outside the medical and scientific fields—especially in the realm commonly referred to as spiritual or religious—have uncovered some intriguing possibilities for harnessing the power of the whole.

Going Beyond the Mind and the Body

This book is not in any way intended to include an exploration of religious traditions and practices. But spiritual questions naturally arise when many patients with a religious orientation begin to take advantage of mind body applications.

The broadest understanding of the placebo effect, which we described as the second major mind body milestone in Chapter 5 (page 71), inherently raises religious questions for many people. Certainly, a religious faith is not necessary to generate the kind of mind body beliefs that can produce healing. But a firm set of spiritual convictions or a strong philosophical worldview can reinforce the intensity of belief associated with effective treatment.

Others of a religious mindset may immediately see the possibility that the innate mind body healing capacities in all humans are "God-given" traits or powers. With this view, learning to exercise these powers may become a natural, if not mandatory, process for those who desire to make the best use of all that they believe God has given them.

The Repetitive Prayer Effect

A factor related specifically to the interaction between spiritual disciplines and mind body healing involves prayer—especially repetitive, meditative prayer.

You will recall that our basic Benson-Henry Protocol, which includes the Phase One triggering of the relaxation response—a protocol firmly established by reductionistic research—features the repetition on each out-breath of what we have called a "focus word" or phrase. That focus may be completely secular and have nothing to do with your worldview. But more often, religious patients prefer to choose a short prayer, passage of Scripture, or other spiritually meaningful utterance. That choice enhances their belief in the mind body healing process and also tends to give them the motivation or "staying power" to persevere with the treatment program on a long-term basis.

A similar spiritual linkage may be established in Phase Two visualization. Instead of a generally pleasant but neutral scene or a random memory of past wellness, the religious patient may create a mental image that includes reassuring spiritual imagery. For example, one Christian patient who chose as her focus the first line from Psalm 23, "The Lord is my shepherd," pictured the ancient statue of Jesus carrying a lamb over his shoulder. This mental picture helped reinforce her belief that the power of God lay behind her mind body practice.

In these ways, mind body healing can merge with—or be bolstered by—religious faith as the patient's faith enhances the power of the patient's expectation-belief.

A Religion-Emergence Link?

These spiritual variations of mind body healing and the synergism between spiritual factors and scientifically established mind body effects may very well be tapping into the emergence phenomenon described earlier. We cannot measure any such emergent result with reductionistic tools or technologies. Nor can we even be sure scientifically that "the whole is really greater than the parts" in these situations. But clinical and anecdotal reports suggest that, in many cases, adding a spiritual component can enhance the mind body healing potential.

One sign of emergence in spirituality is a common principle found in many meditative religious traditions: To experience the full impact of contemplation, prayer, worship, or another spiritual discipline, it is necessary to "let go," "back off," "surrender," or "submit to God." Spiritually, this deferential, passive attitude places God or the Superior Being first and subordinates the human will, with all its anxieties and uncertainties. Physiologically, "letting go" breaks the connection of the body and mind with unproductive, stressful thought patterns and responses and opens the door to the relaxation response and all the healing potential that it can provide.[10]

What are the implications of these spiritual insights for the principles of mind body healing?

At the very least, when such emergent spiritual beliefs and insights are linked to what we know about the relaxation response, the placebo effect, and other mind body phenomena, the healing potential may intensify. Suppose, for instance, that a person who believes in the power of a particular spiritual tradition chooses to incorporate elements of that tradition into Phase One focus words or Phase Two visualizations. In such a situation, the intensity of belief in the procedure—and the physiologic healing power of that belief—will typically increase. The spiritual element may add a component to healing that is incapable of being measured reductionistically and that may, for all we know, be even more powerful than the mind body forces we can measure.

A growing body of scientific literature supports an association between spirituality and good health. An array of research articles and recent reviews in medical journals report that frequent involvement in worship, prayer, and other religious disciplines may promote such signs of health and healthful behavior as these:[11]

- Longevity
- Abstinence from alcohol and smoking
- Lower rates of depression
- Subjective feelings of well-being
- Lower involvement in crime, delinquency, and excessive sexual behaviors
- Higher grade point averages

Our reductionistic research methodology may never establish a definitive, causal relationship between religious commitment and good health or health-inducing behaviors, but that doesn't mean that such a relationship does not exist. We can say only that we currently lack the research tools and the scientific understanding needed to comprehend the relationships. Further, we must recognize that if we are dealing with a genuinely emergent phenomenon as far as human spirituality is concerned, our research tools may never enable us to provide a reductionist, scientific explanation.

Many of the deeper areas of life, then, may enhance healing, even though they cannot be analyzed. The more we probe the most sweeping philosophical questions *and* the minutiae of our molecular and genetic activity, the more we realize that *both reductionism and emergence are essential to our health.* Some areas of inquiry will probably always lie beyond our scientific capacities, just out of our intellectual reach, in the inscrutable realm of emergence and synergism. But those enigmatic regions of reality may still play a significant role in our ability to achieve whole, healthy bodies and minds.

10.

The Future of the Revolution

In this era of deep concern over health care and costs, the question naturally arises: What relevance does mind body medicine have to the social and medical challenges we now face? And what direction can we expect the Relaxation Revolution to take in the future?

In addition to the treatment options described in this book, there appear to be at least three areas where mind body approaches can have a major impact: preventive medicine programs; educational initiatives designed to promote better health habits among young people; and significant cost savings, as mind body treatments become the third major approach to medicine, after drugs and surgery.

The Promise of Preventive Medicine

We have devoted most of the practical application sections of this book to the issue of medical treatment. That is, our suggested mind body approaches have been presented as responses to diseases or medical conditions that already exist in a patient. But there have also been references to using mind body strategies for the *prevention of disease,* and that is the emphasis we want to leave with you now. Every treatment suggested in Chapter 7 (page 109) and elsewhere can be used as part of a prevention plan to head off diseases for which you feel you may be at risk, either because of your personal medical examinations or your family medical history.

Assume you have been diagnosed with borderline high blood pressure, say 135/85 mm Hg. Your physician may have suggested that you try some lifestyle changes to bring those readings down without having to make immediate use of medication. So, following his instructions, you may have altered your diet to lose weight, reduced your salt intake, and increased your aerobic (endurance) exercise.

But you don't have to limit your preventive lifestyle adjustments to these measures. You should consider employing the mind body strategies for treating hypertension suggested in Chapter 7 (page 128). Even though you don't yet have full-blown hypertension, you are well on your way to trouble, and the two-phase protocol we have suggested may help head off the disease and avoid a regimen of antihypertensive pills.

Or let's suppose that you have a family history of heart disease, perhaps with one or both of your parents having suffered heart attacks at a relatively early age. In that case, you should be taking preventive measures to reduce your risk of succumbing to your adverse family history. Your physician may prescribe a number of lifestyle changes, such as losing weight, adjusting your diet so as to reduce your intake of fatty or high-cholesterol foods, stopping smoking, and increasing your regular aerobic exercise. She may also prescribe low doses of a cholesterol-lowering drug if your cholesterol and blood lipid levels remain too high despite dietary changes.

In addition, you should add our two-phase mind body protocol to your preventive plan, perhaps using the suggested approach for lowering PVCs (skipped or extra heartbeats) in Chapter 7 (page 190). Our research and clinical experience have shown that a program incorporating the elicitation of the relaxation response and expectation-belief through visualization can help you treat a number of heart-related problems, and the same benefits apply to prevention of those problems.

But even as we make these recommendations, we must remind you to prepare to deal with a special challenge that plagues most preventive medicine programs, as well as the mind body treatments suggested in these pages: the issue of *time*.

The Challenge of Time

Most preventive medicine programs work well in mitigating, delaying, or completely averting the onset of disease. But most of these programs also require time, effort, and motivation to achieve their full effect. In contrast, Western medicine has accustomed us to the quick fix of taking a pill or submitting to a particular surgery or other procedure to correct a particular health problem. The idea of spending a little time—a solution that may cost little or nothing (except perhaps the onetime cost of being trained in a preventive technique), that carries no negative side effects, and that contributes to total body health and well-being—somehow lacks appeal.

True, our two-phase Benson-Henry Protocol, which encompasses both mind body treatments of diseases and preventive medicine techniques, does take some time and motivation. As we have repeated many times throughout this book, we recommend that you spend 12 to 15 minutes daily in Phase One eliciting the relaxation response and 8 to 10 minutes daily in Phase Two visualization. This mind body total of 20 to 25 minutes will certainly involve more time than taking a pill, but rational analysis and the overwhelming body of scientific literature show clearly that a mind body approach is more than worth the time recommended.

The Educational Opportunity

A natural outgrowth of the preventive use of mind body approaches is to focus on educating young people in the techniques that we describe. Logically, what works for adults should also work for children and teenagers. If they start employing these techniques at a young age, they should be in a much stronger position not only to self-treat themselves for diseases they already have, but also to prevent other diseases in the future.

In 1989, Marilyn Wilcher, senior director of the Benson-Henry Institute, implemented these principles by creating and establishing the Educational Initiative. In 1994 we conducted a study of sophomore students at a high school in Lake Placid, New York.[1] Using a randomized, crossover experimental design for the study, we divided the sophomores into two groups and exposed one of the groups in the fall semester to a health curriculum based on elicitation of the relaxation response, plus a follow-up period to see whether healthful changes persisted. We exposed the second group to a control health curriculum in the fall semester and then to the relaxation response curriculum in the spring semester.

In the relaxation response curriculum, each of the classroom sessions, which were held three times weekly, began with the group's eliciting the relaxation response for 15 minutes (the equivalent of Phase One of our protocol). The students were also encouraged to practice the technique in abbreviated form throughout the day when they encountered anxiety-provoking situations. (This short version of Phase One, what we call a "mini," is described in the box in Chapter 7, page 116, and typically requires 15 seconds or less.) The curriculum included education in stress management, self-esteem, nutrition, drug use, and human sexuality.

To evaluate the results, we arranged for both psychological and physiological testing. On the psychological level, we tested the students' self-esteem and "locus of self-control," or their ability to internalize their self-control, including the management or elimination of inappropriate classroom behavior. On the physical plane, we monitored heart rate and blood pressure.

We concluded that exposure to the relaxation response curriculum resulted in significant increases in self-esteem and a tendency toward a greater internal locus of control—and fewer inappropriate classroom behaviors. In addition, we found a significant reduction in both systolic and diastolic blood pressures as a result of the relaxation response intervention. The students improved both their psychological and physical status as a result of Phase One of the protocol.

In another study we conducted a few years later, in 2000, we found that students at the Horace Mann Middle School in South Central Los Angeles experienced additional benefits as a result of a relaxation response curriculum.[2] Those who had attended more than two semester-long classes, in which teachers had been trained to teach the relaxation response technique, had higher grade point averages, better work habits, and higher levels of cooperation than did students who attended two or fewer such classes. In general, students who had more exposure to the relaxation response curriculum showed an improvement in their academic scores over a two-year period.

Our Educational Initiative brings relaxation response–based coping skills and life management tools into various school environments to help both teachers and students manage their daily stress better and also to improve students' academic performance and health. The program incorporates many of the principles and techniques you have learned, including stress awareness, relaxation response exercises, and visualization.[3]

A Solution to the Challenge of Medical Costs?

When a patient has learned the basic technique for applying mind body approaches in medical treatment and prevention, the technique costs nothing to administer. Ironically, this reality has been one of the major factors operating against the incorporation of mind body techniques into standard medical treatment. There is simply no profit in the field of mind body medicine for drug companies and surgical supply companies, and so they ignore the possibilities of this field of medicine.

Also, teaching a patient a mind body technique and then monitoring the person in the use of that technique takes time—more time than that required to prescribe a pill or even perform a short surgical procedure. Time is money with doctors, as with other professionals. So the physician may be tempted to choose the quick, but expensive, medical fix rather than a perfectly effective procedure that requires more time but may cost considerably less and have fewer side effects.

Unfortunately, this systemic resistance to mind body medicine constitutes a major roadblock to reducing our overall health costs. If we could lower the incidence of disease through effective preventive medicine techniques and also cut costs with less expensive mind body approaches, we might save hundreds of billions of dollars now spent or lost through excessive medications, stress-related diseases, and lost workdays. According to a 2005 article in *Harvard Business Review,* American businesses lose $300 billion each year to reduced productivity, absenteeism, health-care expenses, and related costs that arise from stress.[4]

Other findings bolster these conclusions about the lower-cost potential for mind body medicine. We spend at least $15 billion per year on medications for insomnia alone, which do not work well over the long term and which can often be replaced by mind body interventions.[5] Also, we found in a 1991 study that patient visits to clinics in one year were reduced by 36 percent by our intervention programs.[6] Another study found that a "multimodal behavioral program"—which included such components as physical and occupational therapy, cognitive restructuring, behavioral modification, and relaxation-biofeedback training—resulted in a 58 percent reduction in medical costs.[7]

Unnecessary surgery presents a huge cost problem as well. As mentioned in Chapter 5 (page 72) and Chapter 7 (page 165), billions of dollars are spent annually on unnecessary knee surgery for osteoarthritis. Yet "sham surgery"—fake surgery that patients *believe* is real surgery—is equal or superior to routine surgery because of the power of expectation-belief in treating disease.[8]

Back surgery, too, may be problematic. The estimated annual expenditures for fractures caused by osteoporosis in the United States range from $12 billion to $18 billion in 2002.[9] But research has shown that vertebroplasty—the injection of special cement into the spine, which is a common treatment for this type of fracture—works no better than a "sham" placebo surgery (see Chapter 7, page 150).

The cost of treatment for arthritis is another expense that may be lowered by nondrug, nonsurgical approaches. One study showed a 43 percent reduction in physician visits by arthritis patients who participated in one self-management program,[10] and a 20 to 36 percent decline in medical costs for Medicaid patients who underwent brief psychotherapy treatments for 6 to 12 months.[11] Those Medicaid patients who spent the most time in counseling tended to have the highest-percentage reduction in their medical costs.

A large part of these cost savings with mind body approaches to treatment is probably due to the better management of stress in patients. Researchers have estimated that between 60 and 90 percent of all visits to physicians are largely due to psychological, emotional, and behavioral factors.[12] Of course, mind body treatments deal directly with this stress factor.

The huge amount of money at stake in medical care must not be minimized. An estimated $2.5 trillion is spent every year on health care in the United States, a sum that represents almost one-fifth of the American economy.[13] Imagine the savings that we may achieve as we begin to take the mind body option more seriously. Whatever form of health-care system evolves in the United States, the use of mind body medicine approaches will decrease overall usage of medical services and, concomitantly, reduce medical costs.

Clearly, then, the future of mind body medicine is bright. We have every reason to believe that, with the great progress in research, treatments involving the relaxation response, expectation-belief, and the use of visualization, desensitization, and other cognitive strategies will spread from the medical research laboratories into the patient examining rooms. As the absence of side effects and the lower cost of treatments become obvious, the mind body revolution should accelerate.

We have entirely too much to lose in terms of excessive costs and impaired personal health if we try to stand in the way of this revolution. Yet we have so much to gain if we just accept the scientifically proven fact that the mind can indeed influence and heal the body.

As for you personally, you have the capacity to change your physiology, biochemistry, brain activity, and genetic expression for the better. Isn't it time for you to invest a short period each day to capitalize on your innate and underutilized gifts of healing?

Notes

Chapter 1: The Making of a Revolution

1. Lazar, S. W., G. Bush, R. L. Gollub, G. L. Fricchione, G. Khalsa, and H. Benson, "Functional Brain Mapping of the Relaxation Response and Meditation," *NeuroReport* 11 (2000): 1581–85.

2. Benson, H., and R. Friedman, "Harnessing the Power of the Placebo Effect and Renaming It 'Remembered Wellness,'" *Annual Reviews of Medicine* 47 (1996): 193–99.

3. See also Benson, H., *Timeless Healing* (New York: Scribner, 1996), 146–48, 228–29.

4. Dusek, J. A., H. H. Otu, A. L. Wohlhueter, M. Bhasin, L. F. Zerbini, M. G. Joseph, H. Benson, and T. A. Libermann, "Genomic Counter-Stress Changes Induced by the Relaxation Response," *PLoS ONE*, Jul. 2008, 3(7): e2576, www.plosone.org.

Chapter 2: The Genetic Breakthrough—Your Ultimate Mind Body Connection

1. Dusek et al., "Genomic Counter-Stress Changes Induced by the Relaxation Response," e2576.

2. *Ibid.* Lee, N. H., and A. Saeed, "Microarrays: An Overview," *Methods in Molecular Biology* 353 (2007): 265–300.

3. Zieker, J., D. Dieker, A. Jatzko, J. Dietzsch, K. Nieselt, et al., "Differential Gene Expression in Peripheral Blood of Patients Suffering from Post-traumatic Stress Disorder," *Molecular Psychiatry* 12 (2007): 116–18.

4. The disk, which our scientists called the "Olivia CD," was created by Olivia Ames Hoblitzelle when she was an associate at the Mind/Body Medical Institute. If you are interested in ordering the CD, which is titled *Bring Relaxation to Your Life,* by Olivia Hoblitzelle, please visit our website, www.massgeneral.org/bhi, and click on the link to the "Online Store."

5. Quackenbush, J., "Microarray Analysis and Tumor Classification," *New England Journal of Medicine,* Jun. 8, 2006, 354: 2463–72.

6. Bhasin, M., J. Dusek, B.-H. Chang, G. Fricchione, H. Benson, and T. Libermann, "Genomic Changes Induced by the Relaxation Response Counter Genomic Dysregulation of Several Cancers." Oral presentation at the Society for Integrative Oncology, 6th International Conference, November 12, 2009, New York, NY.

Chapter 3: The Fall and Rise of the Healing Mind

1. For the explanation of how gene expression works to heal, see Chapter 2.

2. Porter, R., *The Greatest Benefit to Mankind: A Medical History of Humanity* (New York: W. W. Norton & Co., 1997, 1998), 230.

3. McGrew, R. E., *Encyclopedia of Medical History* (New York: McGraw-Hill Co., 1985), 298–99. Kennedy, M. T., *A Brief History of Disease, Science & Medicine: From the Ice Age to the Genome Project* (Mission Viejo, CA: Asklepiad Press, 2004), 10, 104.

4. Porter, *The Greatest Benefit to Mankind,* 294–96. McGrew, *Encyclopedia of Medical History,* 312. Kennedy, *A Brief History of Disease, Science & Medicine,* 116–17, 291.

5. *Ibid.*

6. Komaroff, A. L., editor in chief, *Harvard Medical School Family Health Guide* (New York: Free Press, 1999, 2005), 877.

7. *Ibid.*

8. McGrew, *Encyclopedia of Medical History,* 155.

9. Kennedy, *A Brief History of Disease, Science & Medicine,* 111. Porter, *The Greatest Benefit to Mankind,* 277.

10. Porter, *The Greatest Benefit to Mankind*, 433. McGrew, *Encyclopedia of Medical History*, 27–28.

11. McGrew, *Encyclopedia of Medical History*, 27.

12. Porter, *The Greatest Benefit to Mankind*, 434.

13. *Ibid.*, 435.

14. *Ibid.*, 370ff.

15. *Ibid.*, 371. McGrew, *Encyclopedia of Medical History*, 22.

16. Porter, *The Greatest Benefit to Mankind*, 371.

17. *Ibid.*, 404, 436ff. McGrew, 63.

18. Komaroff, *Harvard Medical School Family Health Guide*, 948.

19. Lax, E., *The Mold in Florey's Coat: The Story of the Penicillin Miracle* (New York: Henry Holt and Company, 2005), 1–7, 260–63.

20. Komaroff, *Harvard Medical School Family Health Guide*, 504–5.

21. Chaucer, Geoffrey, *The Canterbury Tales: A Complete Translation into Modern English by Ronald L. Ecker and Eugene J. Crook*, "The Merchant's Tale," lines 1495–1500, Books Online, http://www.ronaldecker.com/merchant.htm.

22. Stefano, G. B., G. L. Fricchione, B. T. Slingsby, and H. Benson, "The Placebo Effect and Relaxation Response: Neural Processes and Their Coupling to Constitutive Nitric Oxide," *Brain Research Reviews* 35 (2001): 2.

23. Inglis, B., *Fringe Medicine* (London: Faber and Faber, 1964), 34–37.

24. This point will become clear as the overwhelming body of evidence showing the positive health impact of belief and expectation is presented in Chapter 5 and in Part II.

25. The following historical material on mind body developments comes from several sources, including the following: Taylor, E. I., *Harvard Medical Alumni Bulletin*, Winter 2000, 40–47. Harrington, A., *The Cure Within: A History of Mind-Body Medicine* (New York: W. W. Norton & Company, Inc., 2008), 91, 110, 123, 144–48, 151, 216. Porter, *The Greatest Benefit to Mankind*, 340, 369, 562, 565, 606, 680.

26. Bryan, C. S., and S. H. Podolsky, "Dr. Holmes at 200—the Spirit of Skepticism," *New England Journal of Medicine*, Aug. 17, 2009, 351(9): 846–47.

27. James, W., *The Varieties of Religious Experience* (New York: The Modern Library, Random House, 1902, 1929), 93–94. See also the commentary in Harrington, *The Cure Within,* 117.

28. Taylor, E. I., *Harvard Medical Alumni Bulletin,* Winter 2000, 44.

29. Harrington, *The Cure Within,* 145.

30. Porter, *The Greatest Benefit to Mankind,* 562.

31. Selye, H., *Stress* (Montreal: Acta, 1950).

32. Harrington, *The Cure Within,* 110.

33. *Ibid.,* 216.

Chapter 4: The Mind Body Milestones—# 1: The Relaxation Response

1. See Stefano et al., "The Placebo Effect," 3; Benson, H., and W. Proctor, *The Breakout Principle* (New York: Scribner, 2003, 2004), 52–53; Benson, H., J. F. Beary, and M. P. Carol, "The Relaxation Response," *Psychiatry,* Feb. 1974, 37: 37–46; and Benson, H., *The Relaxation Response* (New York: Avon, 1976), 25–26.

2. Wallace, R. K., H. Benson, and A. F. Wilson, "A Wakeful Hypometabolic Physiologic State," *American Journal of Physiology,* Sept. 1971, 221(3): 795–99.

3. Benson et al., "The Relaxation Response," 37–46.

4. Hoffman, J. W., H. Benson, P. A. Arns, G. L. Stainbrook, L. Landsberg, J. B. Young, and A. Gill, "Reduced Sympathetic Nervous System Responsivity Associated with the Relaxation Response," *Science,* Jan. 8, 1982, 215: 190–92.

5. Stefano et al., "The Placebo Effect," 9.

6. Dusek, J. A., B.-H. Chang, J. Zaki, S. Lazar, A. Deykin, G. B. Stefano, A. L. Wohlhueter, P. L. Hibberd, and H. Benson, "Association Between Oxygen Consumption and Nitric Oxide Production During the Relaxation Response," *Medical Science Monitor,* Jan. 2006, 12(1): CR1–CR10.

7. Lazar, S. W., C. E. Kerr, R. H. Wasserman, J. R. Gray, D. N. Greve, M. T. Treadway, M. McGarvey, B. T. Quinn, J. A. Dusek, H. Benson, S. L. Rauch, C. I. Moore, and B. Fischl, "Meditation Experience Is Associated with Increased Cortical Thickness," *NeuroReport,* Nov. 28, 2005, 16(17): 1893–97.

8.   Dusek et al., "Genomic Counter-Stress Changes Induced by the Relaxation Response," e2576.

9.   Friedman, R., P. Zuttermeister, and H. Benson, "Correspondence: Unconventional Medicine., *The New England Journal of Medicine*, Oct. 14, 1993, 329(16): 1200–1204.

10. Benson, H., J. A. Herd, W. H. Morse, and R. T. Kelleher, "Behavioral Induction of Arterial Hypertension and Its Reversal," *American Journal of Physiology*, Jul. 1969, 217(1): 30–34.

11. Gutmann, M. C., and H. Benson, "Interaction of Environmental Factors and Systemic Arterial Blood Pressure: A Review," *Medicine*, Nov. 1971, 50(6): 543–53.

12. Benson, H., D. Shapiro, B. Tursky, and G. E. Schwartz, "Decreased Systolic Blood Pressure through Operant Conditioning Techniques in Patients with Essential Hypertension," *Science*, Aug. 1971, 173: 740–43.

13. Benson, H., B. A. Rosner, B. R. Marzetta, and H. M. Klemchuk, "Decreased Blood-Pressure in Pharmacologically Treated Hypertensive Patients Who Regularly Elicited the Relaxation Response," *The Lancet*, Feb. 23, 1974, i: 289–91.

14. Dusek, J. A., P. L. Hibberd, B. Buczynski, B.-H. Chang, K. C. Dusek, J. M. Johnston, A. L. Wohlhueter, H. Benson, and R. M. Zusman, "Stress Management versus Lifestyle Modification on Systolic Hypertension and Medication Elimination: A Randomized Trial," *The Journal of Alternative and Complementary Medicine*, Mar. 1, 2008, 14(2): 129–38.

15. Jacobs, G. D., P. A. Rosenberg, R. Friedman, J. Matheson, G. M. Peavy, A. C. Domar, and H. Benson, "Multifactor Behavioral Treatment of Chronic Sleep-Onset Insomnia Using Stimulus Control and the Relaxation Response," *Behavior Modification*, Oct. 1993, 17(4): 498–509.

16. Jacobs, G. D., H. Benson, and R. Friedman, "Perceived Benefits in a Behavioral-Medicine Insomnia Program: A Clinical Report," *The American Journal of Medicine*, Feb. 1996, 100: 212–16.

17. Benson, H., S. Alexander, and C. L. Feldman, "Decreased Premature Ventricular Contractions through Use of the Relaxation Response

in Patients with Stable Ischaemic Heart-Disease," *The Lancet,* Aug. 30, 1975, 380–86.

18. Komaroff, *Harvard Medical School Family Health Guide,* 1046–47.

19. *Ibid.,* 1047.

20. Goodale, I. L., A. D. Domar, and H. Benson, "Alleviation of Premenstrual Syndrome Symptoms with the Relaxation Response," *Obstetrics & Gynecology,* Apr. 1990, 75(4): 649–55.

21. Komaroff, *Harvard Medical School Family Health Guide,* 90, 907.

22. Domar, A. D., M. M. Seibel, and H. Benson, "The Mind/Body Program for Infertility: A New Behavioral Treatment Approach for Women with Infertility," *Fertility and Sterility,* Feb. 1990, 53(2): 246–49.

Chapter 5: The Mind Body Milestones— # 2: Expectation-Belief

1. Shakespeare, W. *Troilus and Cressida,* III, ii (17).

2. Bacon, F. *Of Truth: Essays* (1625) (The Essays or Counsels, Civil and Moral of Francis Ld. Verulam Viscount St. Albans). Project Gutenberg online text. http://www.gutenberg.org/dirs/etext96/ebacn10.txt.

3. Moseley, J. G., K. O'Malley, N. J. Petersen, T. J. Menke, B. A. Brody, D. H. Kuykendall, J. C. Hollingsworth, C. M. Ashton, and N. P. Wray, "A Controlled Trial of Arthroscopic Surgery for Osteoarthritis of the Knee," *New England Journal of Medicine,* Jul. 11, 2002, 347(2): 81–88.

4. Benson, H., and M. D. Epstein, "The Placebo Effect: A Neglected Asset in the Care of Patients," *Journal of the American Medical Association,* Jun. 23, 1975, 232: 1225–26.

5. Fricchione, G., and G. B. Stefano, "Placebo Neural Systems: Nitric Oxide, Morphine and the Dopamine Brain Reward and Motivation Circuitries," *Medical Science Monitor,* May 2005, 11(5): MS54–65. Epub Apr. 28, 2005. Stefano et al., "The Placebo Effect," 1–19.

6. Benedetti, F., A. Pollo, L. Lopiano, M. Lanotte, S. Vighetti, and I. Rainero, "Conscious Expectation and Unconscious Conditioning in Analgesic, Motor, and Hormonal Placebo-Nocebo Responses," *The Journal of Neuroscience,* May 15, 2003, 23(10): 4315–23.

7.   Benedetti, F., H. S. Mayberg, R. D. Wager, C. S. Stohler, and J.-K. Zubieta, "Neurobiological Mechanisms of the Placebo Effect," *The Journal of Neuroscience,* Nov. 9, 2005, 25(45): 10390–402.

8.   Benson, H., and D. P. McCallie, Jr., "Angina Pectoris and the Placebo Effect," *New England Journal of Medicine* 300 (1979): 1424–29.

9.   http://vsearch.nlm.nih.gov/vivisimo/cgi-bin/query-meta?v%3 Aproject=medlineplus&query=depression.

10. Diederich, N. J., and C. G. Goetz, "The Placebo Treatments in Neurosciences: New Insights from Clinical and Neuroimaging Studies," *Neurology,* Aug. 26, 2008, 71(9): 677–84.

11. *Ibid.*

12. Vallance, A. K., "A Systematic Review Comparing the Functional Neuroanatomy of Patients with Depression Who Respond to Placebo to Those Who Recover Spontaneously: Is There a Biological Basis for the Placebo Effect in Depression?" *Journal of Affective Disorders,* Feb. 2007, 98(1–2): 177–85. Epub Sept. 6, 2006.

13. Alexopoulos, G. S., D. Kanellopoulos, C. Murphy, F. Gunning-Dixon, R. Katz, and M. Heo, "Placebo Response and Antidepressant Response," *American Journal of Geriatric Psychiatry,* Feb. 2007, 15(2): 149–58. Stein, D. J., D. S. Baldwin, O. T. Dolberg, N. Despiegel, and B. Bandelow, "Which Factors Predict Placebo Response in Anxiety Disorders and Major Depression? An Analysis of Placebo-Controlled Studies of Escitalopram," *Journal of Clinical Psychiatry,* Nov. 2006, 67(11): 1741–46.

14. Khan, A., N. Redding, and W. A. Brown, "The Persistence of the Placebo Response in Antidepressant Clinical Trials," *Journal of Psychiatric Research,* Aug. 2008, 42(10): 791–96. Epub Nov. 26, 2007.

15. Stice, E., E. Burton, S. K. Bearman, and P. Rohde, "Randomized Trial of a Brief Depression Prevention Program: An Elusive Search for a Psychosocial Placebo Control Condition," *Behaviour Research and Therapy,* May 2007, 45(5): 863–76. Epub Sept. 27, 2006.

16. Smith, S., C. Anderson-Hanley, A. Langrock, and B. Compas, "The Effects of Journaling for Women with Newly Diagnosed Breast Cancer," *Psychooncology,* Dec. 2005, 14(12): 1075–82.

17.　Fuente-Fernández, R., T. J. Ruth, V. Sossi, M. Schutzer, D. B. Calne, and A. J. Stoessl, "Expectation and Dopamine Release: Mechanism of the Placebo Effect in Parkinson's Disease," *Science* 293 (2001): 1164–66.

18.　Benedetti, F., A. Pollo, L. Lopiano, M. Lanotte, S. Vighetti, and I. Rainero, "Conscious Expectation and Unconscious Conditioning in Analgesic, Motor, and Hormonal Placebo-Nocebo Responses," *The Journal of Neuroscience*, May 15, 2003, 23(10): 4315–23. Benedetti, F., H. S. Mayberg, R. D. Wager, C. S. Stohler, and J.-K. Zubieta, "Neurobiological Mechanisms of the Placebo Effect," *The Journal of Neuroscience*, Nov. 9, 2005, 25(45): 10390–402.

19.　McRae, C., E. Cherin, T. G. Yamazaki, G. Diem, A. H. Vo, D. Russell, J. H. Ellgring, S. Fahn, P. Greene, S. Dillon, H. Winfield, K. B. Bjugstad, and C. R. Freed, "Effects of Perceived Treatment on Quality of Life and Medical Outcomes in a Double-Blind Placebo Surgery Trial," *Archives of General Psychiatry*, 2004, 61: 412–20.

Chapter 6: Planning Your Personal Mind Body Health Strategy

1.　Cooper, K. H., T. C. Cooper, and W. Proctor, *Start Strong, Finish Strong: Prescriptions for a Lifetime of Great Health* (New York: Avery Penguin Group, 2007, 2008), 74.

2.　Lazar et al., "Functional Brain Mapping of the Relaxation Response and Meditation," *NeuroReport*, May 15, 2000, 11(7): 1581–85.

3.　Benson and Friedman, "Harnessing the Power of the Placebo Effect," 193–99. See also Benson, H., and M. D. Epstein, "The Placebo Effect: A Neglected Asset in the Care of Patients," *Journal of the American Medical Association*, Jun. 23, 1975, 232(12): 1225–27.

4.　Benson and Friedman, "Harnessing the Power of the Placebo Effect," 193–99.

Chapter 7: A Guide to Specific Mind Body Treatments

1.　Komaroff, *Harvard Medical School Family Health Guide*, 657–58.

2.　Benson and McCallie, "Angina Pectoris and the Placebo Effect," 1424–29.

3. Weihrauch, T. R., and T. C. Gauler, "Placebo—Efficacy and Adverse Effects in Controlled Clinical Trials," *Arzneimittelforschung,* May 1999, 49(5): 385–93.

4. Van Dixhoorn, J., and A. White, "Relaxation Therapy for Rehabilitation and Prevention in Ischaemic Heart Disease: A Systematic Review and Meta-analysis," *European Journal of Cardiovascular Prevention and Rehabilitation,* Jun. 2005, 12(3): 193–202.

5. For an in-depth discussion of the following symptoms and standard medical treatments, see Komaroff, *Harvard Medical School Family Health Guide,* 172–73, 402–6.

6. *Ibid.,* 405.

7. *Ibid.,* 404, 405, 406.

8. Samuelson, M., M. Foret, M. Baim, J. Lerner, G. Fricchione, H. Benson, J. Dusek, and A. Yeung, "Exploring the Effectiveness of a Comprehensive Mind Body Intervention for Medical Symptom Relief," *Journal of Alternative and Complementary Medicine,* 2010, 16(2): 1–6.

9. Benson, H., F. H. Frankel, R. Apfel, M. D. Daniels, H. E. Schniewind, J. C. Nemiah, P. E. Sifneos, K. D. Crassweller, M. M. Greenwood, J. B. Kotch, P. A. Arns, and B. Rosner, "Treatment of Anxiety: A Comparison of the Usefulness of Self-Hypnosis and a Meditational Relaxation Technique. An Overview," *Psychotherapy and Psychosomatics,* 1978, 30(3–4): 229–42.

10. Carrington, P., G. H. Collings, Jr., H. Benson, H. Robinson, L. W. Wood, P. M. Lehrer, R. L. Woolfork, and J. W. Cole, "The Use of Meditation—Relaxation Techniques for the Management of Stress in a Working Population," *Journal of Occupational Medicine,* Apr. 1980, 22(4): 221–31.

11. Peters, R. K., and H. Benson, "Time Out from Tension," *Harvard Business Review,* Jan.–Feb. 1978, 56(1): 120–24. Peters, R. K., H. Benson, and D. Porter, "Daily Relaxation Response Breaks in a Working Population: 1. Health, Performance and Well-Being," *American Journal of Public Health* 67 (1977): 946–53. Peters, R. K., H. Benson, and J. M. Peters, "Daily Relaxation Response Breaks in a Working Population: 2. Blood Pressure," *American Journal of Public Health* 67 (1977): 954–59.

12. See Benson, H., and Robert Allen, "How Much Stress Is Too Much?" *Harvard Business Review*, Sept.–Oct. 1980, 86–92.

13. See Benson, H., "Stress, Anxiety and the Relaxation Response," *Behavioral and Biological Medicine* 3 (1985): 1–50.

14. http://vsearch.nlm.nih.gov/vivisimo/cgi-bin/query-meta?v%3 Aproject=medlineplus&query=depression.

15. Diederich, N. J., and C. G. Goetz, "The Placebo Treatments in Neurosciences: New Insights from Clinical and Neuroimaging Studies," *Neurology*, Aug. 26, 2008, 71(9): 677–84.

16. Alexopoulos, G. S., D. Kanellopoulos, C. Murphy, F. Gunning-Dixon, R. Katz, and M. Heo, "Placebo Response and Antidepressant Response," *American Journal of Geriatric Psychiatry*, Feb. 2007, 15(2): 149–58. Stein, D. J., D. S. Baldwin, O. T. Dolberg, N. Despiegel, and B. Bandelow, "Which Factors Predict Placebo Response in Anxiety Disorders and Major Depression? An Analysis of Placebo-Controlled Studies of Escitalopram," *Journal of Clinical Psychiatry*, Nov. 2006, 67(11): 1741–46.

17. Khan, A., N. Redding, and W. A. Brown, "The Persistence of the Placebo Response in Antidepressant Clinical Trials," *Journal of Psychiatric Research*, Aug. 2008, 42(10): 791–96. Epub Nov. 26, 2007.

18. *Ibid.*

19. Vallance, A. K., "A Systematic Review Comparing the Functional Neuroanatomy of Patients with Depression Who Respond to Placebo to Those Who Recover Spontaneously: Is There a Biological Basis for the Placebo Effect in Depression?" *Journal of Affective Disorders*, Feb. 2007, 98(1–2): 177–85. Epub Sept. 6, 2006.

20. Stice, E., E. Burton, S. K. Bearman, and P. Rohde, "Randomized Trial of a Brief Depression Prevention Program: An Elusive Search for a Psychosocial Placebo Control Condition," *Behaviour Research and Therapy*, May 2007, 45(5): 863–76. Epub Sept. 27, 2006.

21. Dusek et al., "Association Between Oxygen Consumption and Nitric Oxide Production," CR1–CR10. Stefano et al., "The Placebo Effect and Relaxation Response," 9.

22. For example, see Benson, H., B. A. Rosner, B. R. Marzetta, and H. Klemchuk, "Decreased Blood Pressure in Borderline Hypertensive Subjects Who Practiced Meditation." *Journal of Chronic Diseases* 27 (1974): 163–69. Benson, H., B. A. Rosner, B. R. Marzetta, and H. M. Klemchuk, "Decreased Blood Pressure in Pharmacologically Treated Hypertensive Patients Who Regularly Elicited the Relaxation Response," *The Lancet* (1974): 289–91. Peters et al., "Daily Relaxation Response Breaks in a Working Population: 2. Blood Pressure," 954–59. Stefano et al., "The Placebo Effect and the Relaxation Response," 1–19. Asmar, R., M. Safar, and P. Queneau, "Evaluation of the Placebo Effect and Reproducibility of Blood Pressure Measurement in Hypertension," *American Journal of Hypertension*, Jun. 2001, 14(6 Pt. 1): 546–52.

23. Dusek et al., "Stress Management versus Lifestyle Modification on Systolic Hypertension," 129–38.

24. Komaroff, *Harvard Medical School Family Health Guide*, 90, 903–14.

25. *Ibid.*, 911–12.

26. *Ibid.*, 90.

27. Domar et al., "The Mind/Body Program for Infertility: A New Behavioral Treatment Approach for Women with Infertility," 246–49.

28. Domar, A. D., P. C. Zuttermeister, M. Seibel, and H. Benson, "Psychological Improvement in Infertile Women after Behavioral Treatment: A Replication," *Fertility and Sterility*, Jul. 1992, 58(1): 144–47.

29. Deckro, J. P., A. D. Domar, and R. M. Deckro, "Clinical Application of the Relaxation Response in Women's Health," *AWHONN's Clinical Issues*, 1993, 4(2): 311–19.

30. Jacobs et al., "Multifactor Behavioral Treatment of Chronic Sleep-Onset Insomnia," 498–509.

31. Komaroff, *Harvard Medical School Family Health Guide*, 383.

32. Gangwisch, J. E., S. B. Heymsfield, B. Boden-Albala, R. M. Buijs, F. Kreler, T. G. Pickering, A. G. Rundle, G. K. Zammit, and D. Mala-

spina, "Short Sleep Duration as a Risk Factor for Hypertension: Analyses of the First National Health and Nutrition Examination Survey," *Hypertension,* May 2006, 47(5): 833–39. Epub Apr. 3, 2006.

33. Jacobs et al., "Multifactor Behavioral Treatment of Chronic Sleep-Onset Insomnia," 499. See also Komaroff, *Harvard Medical School Family Health Guide,* 383–85.

34. Komaroff, *Harvard Medical School Family Health Guide,* 384.

35. Samuelson et al., "Exploring the Effectiveness of a Comprehensive Mind Body Intervention," 1–6.

36. Jacobs et al., "Multifactor Behavioral Treatment of Chronic Sleep-Onset Insomnia," 498–509.

37. Jacobs et al., "Perceived Benefits in a Behavioral-Medicine Insomnia Program," 212–16.

38. Jacobs et al., "Multifactor Behavioral Treatment of Chronic Sleep-Onset Insomnia," 498–509.

39. Komaroff, *Harvard Medical School Family Health Guide,* 1047.

40. *Ibid.*

41. Kagan, L., and J. A. Dusek, "Editorial: Mind/Body Interventions for Hot Flashes," *Menopause,* Sept.–Oct. 2006, 13(5): 727–29.

42. Irvin, J. H., A. D. Domar, C. Clark, P. C. Zuttermeister, and R. Friedman, "The Effects of Relaxation Response Training on Menopausal Symptoms," *Journal of Psychosomatic Obstetrics and Gynecology,* 1996, 17: 202–7.

43. Carmody, J., S. Crawford, and L. Churchill, "A Pilot Study of Mindfulness-based Stress Reduction for Hot Flashes," *Menopause,* Sept.–Oct. 2006, 13(5): 760–69.

44. Umland, E. M., "Treatment Strategies for Reducing the Burden of Menopause-Associated Vasomotor Symptoms," *Journal of Managed Care Pharmacy,* Apr. 2008, 14 (Suppl 3): 14–19.

45. Komaroff, *Harvard Medical School Family Health Guide,* 1047–54.

46. Fenlon, D. R., J. L. Corner, and J. S. Haviland, "A Randomized Controlled Trial of Relaxation Training to Reduce Hot Flashes in Women with Primary Breast Cancer," *Journal of Pain Symptom Management,* Apr. 2008, 35(4): 397–405.

47. *Ibid.*

48. Tremblay, A., L. Sheeran, and S. K. Aranda, "Psychoeducational Interventions to Alleviate Hot Flashes: A Systematic Review," *Menopause,* Jan.–Feb. 2008, 15(1): 193–202.

49. Komaroff, *Harvard Medical School Family Health Guide,* 177ff, 254–55.

50. *Ibid.*

51. Samuelson et al., "Exploring the Effectiveness of a Comprehensive Mind Body Intervention," 1–6.

52. Figueroa-Moseley, C., P. Jean-Pierre, J. A. Roscoe, J. L. Ryan, S. Kohli, O. G. Palesh, E. P. Ryan, J. Carroll, and G. R. Morrow, "Behavioral Interventions in Treating Anticipatory Nausea and Vomiting," *Journal of the National Comprehensive Cancer Network,* Jan. 2007, 5(1): 44–50.

53. Yoo, H. J., S. H. Ahn, S. B. Kim, W. K. Kim, and O. S. Han, "Efficacy of Progressive Muscle Relaxation Training and Guided Imagery in Reducing Chemotherapy Side Effects in Patients with Breast Cancer and in Improving Their Quality of Life," *Supportive Care for Cancer,* Oct. 2005, 13(10): 826–33. Epub Apr. 23, 2005.

54. Molassiotis, A., H. P. Yung, B. M. Yam, F. Y. Chan, and T. S. Mok, "The Effectiveness of Progressive Muscle Relaxation Training in Managing Chemotherapy-induced Nausea and Vomiting in Chinese Breast Cancer Patients: A Randomised Controlled Trial," *Supportive Care in Cancer,* Apr. 2002, 10(3): 237–46. Epub Dec. 18, 2001.

55. From the website of the International Association for the Study of Pain, publisher of the journal *Pain,* http://www.iasp-pain.org/AM/Template.cfm?Section=Home&Template=/CM/HTMLDisplay.cfm&ContentID=3058.

56. Sessler, C. N., M. J. Grap, and M. A. Ramsay, "Evaluating and Monitoring Analgesia and Sedation in the Intensive Care Unit," *Critical Care,* 2008, 12 (Suppl 3): S2. Epub May 14, 2008.

57. Komaroff, *Harvard Medical School Family Health Guide,* 381–83.

58. Kabat-Zinn, J., L. Lipworth, and R. Burney, "The Clinical Use of Mindfulness Meditation for the Self-Regulation of Chronic Pain," *Journal of Behavioral Medicine,* Jun. 1985, 8(2): 163–90.

59.   Caudill, M., R. Schnable, P. Zuttermeister, H. Benson, and R. Friedman, "Decreased Clinic Use by Chronic Pain Patients: Response to Behavioral Medicine Intervention," *The Clinical Journal of Pain* 7(1991): 305–10.

60.   Benedetti et al., "Conscious Expectation and Unconscious Conditioning," 4315–23.

61.   Benedetti et al., "Neurobiological Mechanisms of the Placebo Effect," 10390–402.

62.   See Benson and Epstein, "The Placebo Effect," 1225–26; Benedetti et al., "Conscious Expectation and Unconscious Conditioning," 4315–23; Benedetti et al., "Neurobiological Mechanisms of the Placebo Effect," 10390–402; and Fuente-Fernández et al., "Expectation and Dopamine Release," 1164–66.

63.   Buchbinder, R., R. H. Osborne, P. R. Ebeling, J. D. Wark, P. Mitchell, C. Wriedt, S. Graves, M. P. Staples, and B. Murphy, "A Randomized Trial of Vertebroplasty for Painful Osteoporotic Vertebral Fractures," *New England Journal of Medicine*, Aug. 6, 2009, 361(6): 557–68.

64.   Weinstein, J. N., "Balancing Science and Informed Choice in Decisions about Vertebroplasty," *New England Journal of Medicine*, Aug. 6, 2009, 361(6): 619–21.

65.   Buchbinder et al., "A Randomized Trial of Vertebroplasty," 565.

66.   Weinstein, "Balancing Science and Informed Choice in Decisions about Vertebroplasty," 620.

67.   See Caudill et al., "Decreased Clinic Use by Chronic Pain Patients," 305–10.

68.   See Komaroff, *Harvard Medical School Family Health Guide*, 212–51.

69.   *Ibid.*, 627; and Caudill et al., "Decreased Clinic Use by Chronic Pain Patients," 305–10.

70.   See Komaroff, *Harvard Medical School Family Health Guide*, 619ff.

71.   Tei, S., P. L. Faber, D. Lehmann, T. Tsujiuchi, H. Kumano, R. D. Pascual-Marqui, L. R. Gianotti, and K. Kochi, "Meditators and Non-Meditators: EEG Source Imaging During Resting," *Brain Topography*, Nov. 2009, 22(3): 158–65. Marrone, D. F., M. J. Schaner,

B. L. McNaughton, P. F. Worley, and C. A. Barnes, "Immediate-Early Gene Expression at Rest Recapitulates Recent Experience," *Journal of Neuroscience*, Jan. 30, 2008, 28(5): 1030–33. Paquette, V., J. Levesque, B. Mensour, J. M. Leroux, G. Beaudoin, P. Bourgouin, and M. Beauregard, "'Change the Mind and You Change the Brain': Effects of Cognitive Behavioral Therapy on the Neural Correlates of Spider Phobia," *Neuroimage*, Feb. 2003, 18(2): 401–409.

72. See Komaroff, *Harvard Medical School Family Health Guide*, 183–86.

73. Benson, H., H. P. Klemchuk, and J. R. Graham, "The Usefulness of the Relaxation Response in the Therapy of Headache," *Headache*, Apr. 1974, 14(1): 49–52.

74. Benson, H., "The Relaxation Response: How to Lower Blood Pressure, Cope with Pain, and Reduce Anxiety in 20 Minutes a Day," *Harvard Medical Bulletin*, Fall 1986: 35.

75. Caudill et al., "Decreased Clinic Use by Chronic Pain Patients," 305–10.

76. Samuelson et al., "Exploring the Effectiveness of a Comprehensive Mind Body Intervention," 1–6.

77. Benson, H., B. Pomeranz, and I. Kutz, "The Relaxation Response and Pain," *Textbook of Pain—the Relaxation Process* (New York: Churchill Livingstone, 1984), 817–22.

78. Fentress, D. W., B. J. Masek, J. E. Mehegan, and H. Benson, "Biofeedback and Relaxation Response Training in the Treatment of Pediatric Migraine," *Developmental Medicine & Child Neurology*, 1986, 28: 139–46.

79. Tilley, B. C., G. S. Alarcon, S. P. Heyse, D. E. Trenham, R. Neuner, D. A. Kaplan, D. O. Clegg, J. C. Leisen, L. Buckley, S. M. Cooper, H. Duncan, S. R. Pillemer, M. Tuttleman, and S. E. Fowler, "Minocycline in Rheumatoid Arthritis: A 48-Week, Double-Blind, Placebo-Controlled Trial," *Annals of Internal Medicine*, Jan. 15, 1995, 122: 81–89. Traut, E. F., and E. W. Passarelli, "Placebos in the Treatment of Rheumatoid Arthritis and Other Rheumatic Conditions," *Annals of the Rheumatic Diseases*, 1957, 16: 18–22.

80. Komaroff, *Harvard Medical School Family Health Guide,* 218–19, 633–34.

81. Moseley, J. G., K. O'Malley, N. J. Petersen, T. J. Menke, B. A. Brody, D. H. Kuykendall, J. C. Hollingsworth, C. M. Ashton, and N. P. Wray, "A Controlled Trial of Arthroscopic Surgery for Osteoarthritis of the Knee," *New England Journal of Medicine,* Jul. 11, 2002, 347(2): 81–88.

82. Bernstein, J., and T. Quach, "A Perspective on the Study of Moseley et al.: Questioning the Value of Arthroscopic Knee Surgery for Osteoarthritis," *Cleveland Clinic Journal of Medicine,* May 2003, 70(5): 401, 405–6, 408–10.

83. Komaroff, *Harvard Medical School Family Health Guide,* 226–28.

84. Caudill et al., "Decreased Clinic Use by Chronic Pain Patients," 305–10. Caudill, M., *Managing Your Pain Before It Manages You* (New York: The Guilford Press, 3rd edition, 2008).

85. Leserman, J., E. M. Stuart, M. E. Mamish, and H. Benson, "The Efficacy of the Relaxation Response in Preparing for Cardiac Surgery," *Behavioral Medicine,* Fall 1989: 111–17.

86. Domar, A. D., J. M. Noe, and H. Benson, "The Preoperative Use of the Relaxation Response with Ambulatory Surgery Patients," *Journal of Human Stress,* Fall 1987: 101–7.

87. Renzi, C., L. Peticca, and M. Pescatori, "The Use of Relaxation Techniques in the Perioperative Management of Proctological Patients: Preliminary Results," *International Journal of Colorectal Diseases,* Nov. 2000, 15(5–6): 313–16.

88. Benson and Proctor, *The Breakout Principle,* 210–11.

89. Komaroff, *Harvard Medical School Family Health Guide,* 371–73.

90. *Ibid.,* 372.

91. *Ibid.,* 373.

92. Fuente-Fernández et al., "Expectation and Dopamine Release," 1164–66.

93. Benedetti et al., "Conscious Expectation and Unconscious Conditioning," 4315–23. Benedetti et al., "Neurobiological Mechanisms of the Placebo Effect," 10390–402.

94. McRae et al., "Effects of Perceived Treatment on Quality of Life," 412–20.

95. Komaroff, *Harvard Medical School Family Health Guide*, 405–6.

96. Van Ameringen, M., C. Mancini, B. Patterson, and W. Simpson, "Pharmacotherapy for Social Anxiety Disorder: An Update," *Israel Journal of Psychiatry and Related Sciences*, 2009, 46(1): 53–61. Owen, R. T., "Controlled-Release Fluvoxamine in Obsessive-Compulsive Disorder and Social Phobia," *Drugs of Today*, Dec. 2008, 44(12): 887–93. "Understanding Phobias—Treatment." WebMD.com: http://www.webmd.com/anxiety-panic/understanding-phobias-treatment. Bailey, J. E., A. Papadopoulos, A. Lingford-Hughes, and D. J. Nutt, "D-Cycloserine and Performance under Different States of Anxiety in Healthy Volunteers," *Psychopharmacology*, Sept. 2007, 193(4): 579–85. See also Komaroff, *Harvard Medical School Family Health Guide*, 1160–89.

97. Granado, L. C., R. Ranvaud, and J. R. Pelaez, "A Spiderless Arachnophobia Therapy: Comparison between Placebo and Treatment Groups and Six-Month Follow-Up Study," *Neural Plasticity*, 2007: 10241.

98. Komaroff, *Harvard Medical School Family Health Guide*, 406.

99. Greenwood, M. M., and H. Benson, "The Efficacy of Progressive Relaxation in Systematic Desensitization and a Proposal for an Alternative Competitive Response—the Relaxation Response," *Behavioral Research & Therapy* 15(1977): 337–43.

100. Hunt, M., L. Bylsma, J. Brock, M. Fenton, A. Goldberg, R. Miller, T. Tran, and J. Urgelles, "The Role of Imagery in the Maintenance and Treatment of Snake Fear," *Journal of Behavioral Therapy and Experimental Psychiatry*, Dec. 2006, 37(4): 283–98. Epub Feb. 13, 2006.

101. Ost, L. G., U. Sterner, and J. Fellenius, "Applied Tension, Applied Relaxation, and the Combination in the Treatment of Blood Phobia," *Behavioral Research and Therapy*, 1989, 27(2): 109–21.

102. Ditto, B., C. R. France, M. Albert, and N. Byrne, "Dismantling Applied Tension: Mechanisms of a Treatment to Reduce Blood Dona-

tion-related Symptoms," *Transfusion*, Dec. 2007, 47(12): 2217–22. Epub Aug. 21, 2007.

103.   Choy, Y., A. J. Fyer, and J. D. Lipsitz, "Treatment of Specific Phobia in Adults," *Clinical Psychology Review*, Apr. 2007, 27(3): 266–86. Epub Nov. 15, 2006.

104.   Cooper, K. H., T. C. Cooper, and W. Proctor, *Start Strong, Finish Strong: Prescriptions for a Lifetime of Great Health* (New York: Avery, 2007, 2008), 114.

105.   Lazar, S. W., C. E. Kerr, R. H. Wasserman, J. R. Gray, D. N. Greve, M. T. Treadway, M. McGarvey, B. T. Quinn, J. A. Dusek, H. Benson, S. L. Rauch, C. I. Moore, and B. Fischl, "Meditation Experience Is Associated with Increased Cortical Thickness," *NeuroReport*, Nov. 28, 2005, 16(17): 1893–97.

106.   Galvin, J. A., H. Benson, G. R. Deckro, G. L. Fricchione, J. A. Dusek, "The Relaxation Response: Reducing Stress and Improving Cognition in Healthy Aging Adults," *Complementary Therapies in Clinical Practice* 12(2006): 186–91.

107.   Dusek et al., "Genomic Counter-Stress Changes Induced by the Relaxation Response," e2576.

108.   Benson and Proctor, *The Breakout Principle*, 225–27.

109.   For an extensive treatment on heart irregularities, see Komaroff, *Harvard Medical School Family Health Guide*, 672–82.

110.   Samuelson et al., "Exploring the Effectiveness of a Comprehensive Mind Body Intervention for Medical Symptom Relief," 1–6

111.   Benson, Alexander, and Feldman, "Decreased Premature Ventricular Contractions through Use of the Relaxation Response," 380–86.

112.   Hellman, C. J., M. Budd, J. Borysenko, D. C. McClelland, and H. Benson, "A Study of the Effectiveness of Two Group Behavioral Medicine Interventions for Patients with Psychosomatic Complaints," *Behavioral Medicine*, Winter 1990, 16(4): 165–73.

113.   Valente, S. M., "Diagnosis and Treatment of Panic Disorder and Generalized Anxiety in Primary Care," *Nurse Practitioner*, Aug. 1996, 21(8): 26, 32–34, 37–38, *passim*.

114.   Komaroff, *Harvard Medical School Family Health Guide*, 680.

115. *Ibid.*, 1046–47.

116. *Ibid.*

117. *Ibid.*, 1047.

118. *Ibid.*

119. Goodale, I. L., A. D. Domar, and H. Benson, "Alleviation of Premenstrual Syndrome Symptoms with the Relaxation Response," *Obstetrics & Gynecology*, Apr. 1990, 75(4): 649–55.

120. Arias, A. J., K. Steinberg, A. Ganga, and R. L. Trestman, "Systematic Review of the Efficacy of Meditation Techniques as Treatments for Medical Illness," *Journal of Alternative and Complementary Medicine*, Oct. 2006, 12(8): 817–32.

121. Limosin, F., and J. Ades, "Psychiatric and Psychological Aspects of Premenstrual Syndrome," *L'Encéphale*, Nov.–Dec. 2001, 27(6): 501–508.

122. Rapkin, A., "Review of Treatment of Premenstrual Syndrome and Premenstrual Dysphoric Disorder," *Psychoneuroendocrinology*, Aug. 2003, 28 (Suppl 3): 39–53.

123. Dvivedi, J., S. Dvivedi, K. K. Hahajan, S. Mittal, and A. Singhal, "Effect of '61-Points Relaxation Technique' on Stress Parameters in Premenstrual Syndrome," *Indian Journal of Physiology and Pharmacology*, Jan.-Mar. 2008, 52(1): 69–76.

124. See Benson, *Timeless Healing*, 228–29.

Chapter 8: Cancer and the Genetic Horizons of Mind Body Treatment

1. Figueroa-Moseley et al., "Behavioral Interventions in Treating Anticipatory Nausea and Vomiting," 44–50.

2. "Pruritus (PDQ®)—Health Professional Version. Etiology/Pathophysiology," National Cancer Institute, www.cancer.gov.

3. Pogatzki-Zahn, E., M. Marziniak, G. Schneider, T. A. Luger, and S. Stander, "Chronic Pruritus: Targets, Mechanisms and Future Therapies," *Drug News Perspectives*, Dec. 2008, 21(10): 541–51.

4. Dusek et al., "Genomic Counter-Stress Changes Induced by the Relaxation Response," e2576.

5. Bhasin et al., "Genomic Changes Induced by the Relaxation Response."

Chapter 9: The Whole Is Greater Than the Sum of Its Parts

1. Downward, J., "Finding the Weakness in Cancer," *New England Journal of Medicine*, Aug. 27, 2009, 361(9): 922–24.

2. This comment, by M.I.T. science historian Evelyn Fox Keller, was reported in a Nov. 11, 2008, article by Natalie Angier in the *New York Times* ("Scientists and Philosophers Find That 'Gene' Has a Multitude of Meanings").

3. Heng, H. H. Q., "The Conflict between Complex Systems and Reductionism," *The Journal of the American Medical Association*, Oct. 1, 2008, 300(13): 1580–81. Heng cites Gerstein, H. C., M. E. Miller, R. P. Byington et al., "Effects of Intensive Glucose Lowering in Type 2 Diabetes," *New England Journal of Medicine*, Jun. 12, 2008, 358(24): 2545–59.

4. *Ibid.*, 1580–81.

5. Mittra, I., "The Disconnection between Tumor Response and Survival," *National Clinical Practice in Oncology*, Apr. 2007, 4(4): 203. Savage, L., "High-Intensity Chemotherapy Does Not Improve Survival in Small Cell Lung Cancer," *Journal of National Cancer Institute*, 2009, 100: 519. Bear, H. D., "Earlier Chemotherapy for Breast Cancer: Perhaps Too Late but Still Useful," *Annals of Surgical Oncology*, May 2003, 10(4): 334–35.

6. Komaroff, *Harvard Medical School Family Health Guide*, 383–85.

7. Randall, J. H., Jr., *Aristotle* (New York: Columbia University Press, 1960), 206–11. Guthrie, W. K. C., *The Greek Philosophers: From Thales to Aristotle* (New York: Harper Torchbooks, 1950), 144.

8. Cho, Adrian, "Ourselves and Our Interactions: The Ultimate Physics Problem?" *Science*, Jul. 2009, 325: 406–8.

9. Heng, "The Conflict Between Complex Systems and Reductionism," 1580.

10. Benson and Proctor, *The Breakout Principle*, 19, 20, 26ff.

11. McCullough, M. E., and B. L. B. Willoughby, "Religion, Self-Regulation, and Self-Control: Associations, Explanations, and Implications," *Psychological Bulletin*, Jan. 2009, 135(1): 69–93.

Chapter 10: The Future of the Revolution

1. Benson, H., A. Kornhaber, C. Kornhaber, M. N. LeChanu, P. C. Zuttermeister, P. Myers, and R. Friedman, "Increases in Positive Psychological Characteristics with a New Relaxation Response Curriculum in High School Students," *The Journal of Research and Development in Education*, Summer 1994, 27(4): 226–31.

2. Benson, H., M. Wilcher, B. Greenberg, E. Huggins, M. Ennis, P. C. Zuttermeister, P. Myers, and R. Friedman, "Academic Performance among Middle School Students after Exposure to a Relaxation Response Curriculum," *Journal of Research and Development in Education*, 2000, 33(3): 156–65.

3. To learn more about this program, contact Marilyn Wilcher at mwilcher@partners.org or call (617) 643-6035.

4. "Different Voice: Are You Working Too Hard? A Conversation with Mind/Body Researcher Herbert Benson," *Harvard Business Review*, Nov. 2005.

5. R. Friedman, "Proceedings and Debates of the 103rd Congress, Second Session," *Congressional Record*, Jun. 13, 1996, 140(73).

6. Caudill et al., "Decreased Clinic Use by Chronic Pain Patients," 305–10.

7. Simmons, J. W., W. S. Avant, J. Demski, and D. Parisher, "Determining Successful Pain Clinic Treatment through Validation of Cost Effectiveness," *Spine*, Mar. 1988, 13: 342–44.

8. Bernstein et al., "A Perspective on the Study of Moseley et al.: Questioning the Value of Arthroscopic Knee Surgery for Osteoarthritis," 401, 405–6, 408–10. See Moseley et al., "A Controlled Trial of Arthroscopic Surgery for Osteoarthritis of the Knee," 81–88.

9. Weinstein, "Balancing Science and Informed Choice in Decisions about Vertebroplasty," 619–21.

10. Friedman, R., M. Sedler, P. Myers, and H. Benson, "Behavioral Medicine, Complementary Medicine, and Integrated Care: Economic Implications," *Complementary and Alternative Therapies in Primary Care*, Dec. 1997, 24(4): 949–62.

11. Friedman, R., D. Sobel, P. Myers, M. Caudill, and H. Benson, "Be-

havioral Medicine, Clinical Health Psychology, and Cost Offset," *Health Psychology,* Nov. 1995, 14(6): 509–18.

12.   Kroenke, K., and A. D. Mangelsdorff, "Common Symptoms in Ambulatory Care: Incidence, Evaluation, Therapy and Outcome," *American Journal of Medicine,* 1989, 86: 262–66.

13.   Abelson, R., "Policy and Profit: Following the Money in the Health Care Debate," *New York Times,* Jun. 14, 2009, www.nytimes.com.

Index

abdominal pain, 15
abenzodiazepine, 179
ACE (angiotensin converting
    enzyme) inhibitors, 129,
    130
"Adam" (case study), 21–28
adrenaline, xi
aerobic exercise, 96, 186, 226
aging, 168, 188
    premature, 16, 23, 29, 186–90
Agnes (patient), 154–55
AIDS, 44
alcohol, 65, 68, 69, 133, 136, 197
Alexander, Sidney, 192
allergic skin reactions, 16, 200
alternative medicine, 33, 46, 208
American Journal of Physiology, 60
amitriptyline, 124
anesthesia, 175
anger, 16, 169, 200, 208
angina pectoris, 112–17
    mind body treatments for, 15,
        30, 114–17

placebo effect and, 79–81,
    114–15
standard treatment for, 113–14
symptoms of, 112–13
angiotensin-II receptor antagonists,
    129
anthrax, 39, 42
antibiotics, 43–45, 54, 132, 218
antidepressants, 82, 158
    see also selective serotonin
        reuptake inhibitors; *specific
        antidepressants*
antiemetics, 146
antihypertensive medication, 63
antiseptic procedure, 40–41
antitetanus toxin, 43
anxiety, 117–23
    of infertile women, 133
    mind body treatments for, xiii,
        15, 55, 59, 119–22
    phobias and, 179, 180
    PVCs, palpitations and, 195
    standard treatment for, 118–19

anxiety (*cont.*)
  before surgery, 169, 171, 175
  symptoms of, 117–18
anxiety paradox, 122–23
applied tension, 181, 183
Archives of General Psychiatry,
    85–86, 177
Aristotle, 217
arteriogram, 113
arthritis, 72–73, 165, 231
arthroscopic debridement, 72–73,
    165–66
arthroscopic lavage, 72, 165–66
aspirin, 158
assisted reproductive technology, 132
asthma, 16

back pain, xii, 4–15, 27, 154–55
back surgery, 6, 8, 14, 230–31
Bacon, Francis, 71
bacteria, 40, 42, 44
Baylor College of Medicine, 72–73,
    165–66
Behavioral Medicine, 170, 192
behavioral training, 192
Behaviour Research and Therapy, 82,
    126
belief, 56, 70, 71–88, 110, 112, 125,
    178
  angina pectoris countered by,
    79–81
  chronic pain countered by,
    78–79

depression countered by, 81–85,
    87–88, 125–26
  in early medicine, 32–33, 34
  heart-related problems
    countered by, 226
  necessity of, for mind body
    healing, 8
  Parkinson's and, 85–87
  physician's influence on,
    73–74
  reductionism and, 74, 216
  spiritual vs. scientific, 75–76
  see also placebo effect
Benedetti, Fabrizio, 79
Benson, Herbert:
  on blood pressure and
    hypertension, 60–61, 62
  Caroline's work with, 7–9,
    10–15, 27
  on infertility, 69–70
  on insomnia, 66, 137
  on irregular heartbeats, 67–68
  and PMS work, 68–69, 198
  reductionism learned by, 211,
    212–13
  relaxation response break and,
    120
Benson-Henry Institute for Mind
    Body Medicine, xiii, xiv, 7,
    21, 24, 30, 58, 144, 188, 192,
    204, 213, 219, 228
Benson-Henry Protocol, 9–10, 19,
    62, 64, 66, 70, 76, 85, 110

Phase One, *see* relaxation response

Phase Two, *see* visualization

benzodiazepine, 118, 135

beta-blockers, 114, 128, 158, 179

Beth Israel Deaconess Medical Center, xiii–xiv, 17, 21, 133, 170–71

Beth Israel Hospital, 69

Bhasin, Manoj, 205

bibliotherapy, 83–84

biofeedback conditioning techniques, 61, 162, 230

biopsy, 172

bloodletting, 32

blood phobias, 181–82, 183

blood pressure, xii, 22, 56, 101, 219, 228–29

high, *see* hypertension

measurement of, 61*n*

blood transfusions, 218

bradycardia, 191, 193

bradykinesia, 176

brain responses, 157

Breakout Principle, The (Benson and Proctor), 103

breast cancer, 15, 141, 142, 145–46

breath focus, 9, 27, 59, 94, 95, 111, 112, 115, 122–23, 155, 162, 222

breathing, diaphragmatic, 24

breathing rate, 9, 11, 27, 56, 93

Broad Institute, 205

bromocriptine, 132

bronchial asthma, 16, 200

buspirone, 118

caffeine, 65, 68, 136, 191, 197

calcium antagonists, 129

Cameron (patient), 202–4, 205–8

cancer, 202–8, 214

breast, 15, 141, 142, 145–46

genetic characteristics of, 23, 30

oxidative stress and, 23

skin, 170–73

surgery for, 43, 172–73

Cannon, Walter, 48, 49, 51–52, 212

Canterbury Tales, The (Chaucer), 45–46

carbidopa, 176

carbolic acid, 40, 41, 42

cardiac surgery, 170

Carl (patient), 172–73

Caroline (patient), 3–7

relaxation response used by, 7–12, 13, 27

visualization by, 12–15

Carrington, Patricia, 119, 120

Cartesian dualism, 17–18, 22

cataracts, 43

Catherine the Great, Empress of Russia, 37

Caudill, Margaret, 149, 168

chaos, 218

Chaucer, Geoffrey, 45–46

chemotherapy, 145, 202–3, 207, 215
Children's Hospital Boston, 161
cholera, 42
cholesterol, 101, 226
chronic pain, xiii, 30, 48, 55, 78, 87,
    148, 149
cinchona bark, 34
claustrophobia, 179, 182, 183–86
Clinical Psychology Review, 182
clomiphene citrate, 132
cluster headaches, 55, 158–59
cognitive behavioral therapy (CBT),
    83, 84, 106–8
cognitive restructuring, 107
cognitive therapy, 182, 216
cold sores, 16
combination treatment, 79, 92
congestive heart failure, 16, 200
Connecticut Medical School,
    University of, 198
constipation, 16, 200
coronary artery bypass, 114
cortex, 23, 58, 81
cough, 16, 200
cramps, 152, 153

dementia, 178
depression, 123–27
    of infertile women, 133
    mind body treatments for, xiii,
        15, 30, 55, 59, 125–27, 216
    placebo effect and, 48, 81–85,
        87–88, 125–26

standard medical treatment for,
    124–25
symptoms of, 123–24
Descartes, René, 17, 18
desensitization, 107–8, 121
desensitization therapy, 180
diabetes mellitus, 16, 43, 200, 215,
    217
diaries, 83, 84
diphtheria, 42–43
direct actual exposure, 180, 182
disease-based model, 106
disks, back, 4, 5–6
diuretics, 129
dizziness, 16, 200
DNA, 214–15
Domar, Alice, 69–70, 133, 140,
    170–71, 198
dopamine, 176, 177
double-blind controlled research,
    46–48, 86, 214
drowsiness, 16, 200
drugs, xii, xiii, 4, 7, 14, 17, 22, 32, 37,
    39, 52, 53, 56, 73, 74, 80, 92,
    109, 110, 114, 149–50, 225,
    229
drug use, 228
duodenal ulcers, 16, 200
Dusek, Jeffrey, 21, 58, 62–63

Ebert, Robert, 213
echocardiogram, 113
education, 227–29

Educational Initiative, 228–29
electrocardiogram (ECG), 113, 193
electroconvulsive therapy (ECT), 125
emergence, 208, 217, 219–21, 222–24
emotions, 51, 52, 113
endorphins, 79, 126, 150, 152
epidemiology, 49
estrogen, 139
European Journal of Cardiovascular Prevention and Rehabilitation, 115
exercise, 65, 96, 113, 114, 128, 136, 139, 186, 215, 226
exercise ECG, 113
exorcisms, 33
Expectation-Belief Milestone, 54, 76–77
expectations, *see* belief
experience-dependent cortical plasticity, 187–88
expressive writing, 84

fatigue, 16, 158, 163, 200
fats, 226
Feldman, Charles, 192
Fentress, David, 161
Fertility and Sterility, 133
fertility drugs, 132
fight-or-flight response, 4–5, 48, 51–52, 212
    relaxation response vs., xi, 8, 52, 56

Finland, Maxwell, 44
Fleming, Alexander, 43
Florey, Howard, 43
fluoxetine, 124, 125
focus word, focusing, 9, 10, 11, 27, 94, 95, 111, 115, 122–23, 155, 222
    for headaches, 162, 163
folk medicines, 32–33, 37
Foret, Megan, 135, 144
free radicals, 23
Freudians, 52
Fricchione, Gregory, xiv, 58
Friedman, Richard, 66, 137
Fuente-Fernández study, 85, 87, 176–77, 178
full relaxation therapy, 117
functional magnetic resonance imaging (fMRI), xii, 13, 58, 103, 105, 187, 214

gangrene, 40
generalized anxiety disorder, 118
genes, reductionism and, 214–15
genetic response, 10, 20–30, 56, 58
    active control of, xi, xii, 14, 18, 20, 53
    of relaxation response, 10, 24–30, 56, 58–59, 204
    stress and, 23–24, 63–64, 157
germs, 40, 49
global gene expression difference, 22–23

Goodale, Irene, 68–69, 198
Graham, John R., 159
guided imagery and visualization, 180
Gutmann, Mary, 61–62

Harvard Business Review, 120, 230
Harvard Medical School, xiii, 17–18, 21, 49, 57, 60, 69, 168, 170–71, 192, 211–13
Harvard Medical School Family Health Guide, 36, 68, 69, 133, 198
headaches, 15, 59
    cluster, 55, 158–59
    migraine, xii, 55, 158, 159, 160, 161–63
    tension, xii, 158, 160
    visualization for, 158–63
head pain, 15
heart attacks, 16
heartbeats, irregular, *see* premature ventricular contractions (PVCs)
heart disease, oxidative stress and, 23
heart rate, xii, 56, 93, 118, 169, 228
Hellman, C. J., 192
Heng, Henry H. Q., 215, 218
herbs, 32, 33, 142
herniated disk, 154, 156
herpes simplex, 16, 200
heterocyclic antidepressants (HCA), 118, 124, 135

Hippocrates, 33
HIV, 44
Hoblitzelle, Olivia, 98n
Holmes, Oliver Wendell, 49–50, 52
Holmes-Rahe scale, 120–21
Holter monitor, 192, 194
homeostasis, 52
Horace Mann Middle School, 229
hormone replacement therapy, 139, 140, 141
hormones, 132, 157, 196
    see also specific hormones
hostility, 16, 200
hot flashes, xii, 15, 139, 140, 141, 142, 143
human genome sequencing, 214
hypertension, 128–31
    insomnia and, 135
    mind body treatments for, 15, 16, 30, 55, 60–64, 120, 129–31, 216, 226
    nocebo effect and, 189–90
    standard treatment for, 128–29
    symptoms of, 110, 128
Hypertension, 135
hypnosis, 57, 119
hypometabolic physiologic state, 57

idiopathic pains, 6
imipramine, 124
immune system, 16, 23, 29, 43
impotency, 16, 200

infertility, 132–34
  mind body treatments for, 15,
    55, 60, 69–70, 133–34
  standard treatment for, 132–33
  symptoms of, 132
inoculations, 36
insomnia, 134–39
  possible mind body treatment
    for, 15, 55, 59, 60, 64–66,
    135–39, 216
  reductionist treatment for, 215
  standard treatment for, 135
  symptoms of, 134–35
insulin, 43
International Association for the
  Study of Pain, 147
*International Journal of Colorectal
  Diseases,* 173
in vitro fertilization, 132
Irvin, J. H., 140
ischemia, 113, 115
isolated systolic hypertension, 63
Italy, 173–74

Jacobs, Gregg, 64, 66, 136, 137
James, William, 48, 49, 50–51, 52
Jenner, Edward, 36
Jennifer, 183–86
Jesuit bark, 34
journaling, 84
Journal of Human Stress, 170–71
Journal of Managed Care Pharmacy,
  141

Journal of Neuroscience, 78, 79
Journal of Psychiatric Research, 82
*Journal of Psychosomatic Obstetrics
  and Gynecology,* 140
*Journal of the American Medical
  Association,* 215, 218
*Journal of the National
  Comprehensive Cancer
  Network,* 145

Kegel exercises, 139
Keith (patient), 193–97
ketorolac tromethamine, 78, 79
knee pain, 15
Koch, Robert, 38, 40, 41–43, 50, 54
Kripalu yoga, 59
Kundalini yoga, 59

Lancet, 41, 61–62, 66, 192
Lazar, Sara, 58, 103, 187
Leserman, Jane, 170
leukemia, 202–3, 204, 205, 206, 207
levodopa (L-dopa), 86, 178
Lind, James, 34–35
linseed oil, 40
lipids, 226
liposuction, 215
Lister, Joseph, 38, 39, 40–41, 42, 50,
  54
locus of self-control, 228
luteinizing hormone, 132
lymph glands, 42
lymphoma, 205

Index

McCallie, David P., Jr., 79–80, 114
magnetic resonance imaging
 (MRI), 5
malaria, 34
mantras, 25, 59
Massachusetts Medical School,
 University of, 140–41
Massachusetts General Hospital,
 xiii, 17, 51, 63, 103
Matthew Thornton Health Plan, 168
Medicaid, 231
medical costs, xii, 229–31, 232
medicine, modern:
 acceleration of, 37–45
 birth of, 34–37
 mind body techniques rejected
  by, 16–17, 20
 as reductionist, 74, 208, 211–16,
  220, 224
meditation, 20, 57, 58, 59, 62, 96,
 119–20
memory, 110, 112
menopause, 139–43
 mind body approaches to, 15,
  140–43, 198
 standard treatment for, 139–40
 symptoms of, 139
Menopause, 142
mental "body scans," 24–25
mental imagery, 9
 see also visualization
"Merchant's Tale, The" (Chaucer),
 45–46

Merck & Co., 44
metabolism, xii, 56, 93
methylphenidate, 124
microarray analysis, 22–23, 214
microscope, 37, 40
migraine headaches, xii, 55, 158,
 159, 160, 161–63
Miller, Anne, 43
Mind body divide, 17–18, 22
Mind Body Healing Model, 18–19
Mind/Body Medical Institute, xiii,
 21*n*, 159, 213
mind body techniques, 8–9
 in conjunction with
  mainstream medicine, *see*
  drugs; surgery
 genetic expression altered by, 14,
  18, 20–30, 53
 in move into medical
  mainstream, 52–53, 54
 in nineteenth century, 48–52
 origins of, 32–34
 scientific support for, xiii, 3, 8,
  17–18, 19, 20–30, 21*n*, 110,
  180–83, 187–88, 192–93
 skepticism of, 16–17, 20, 73–74
 see also Benson-Henry Protocol;
  placebo effect
mindfulness-based stress-reduction
 program (MBSR), 141
mindfulness meditation, 25, 59, 96
"mini" relaxation response exercise,
 115–16, 228

monoamine oxidase inhibitors
(MAOI), 124–25, 179
multiple myeloma, 205
muscle relaxation, 123
music, 97
repetitive-worship, 20

Napoleon I, Emperor of the French,
35, 37
National Heart, Lung, and Blood
Institute, 91
National Institutes of Health (NIH),
81, 123, 213
National Public Radio, 63
nausea, 118, 144–47, 161, 207
mind body treatments for, 15,
144–47
standard treatment for, 144
symptoms of, 144
neck and shoulder pain, 15, 16,
168–69
nerves, 157
neurons, 157
neuroplasticity, 157
NeuroReport, 103, 187
neurotransmitters, 79, 126, 150, 152,
196
neuro tumors, 205
New England Deaconess Hospital, 69
New England Journal of Medicine,
59, 72, 79–80, 114, 150, 151,
165, 166, 168
nicotine, 65, 69

night sweats, 139, 141, 142
nitric oxide (NO), xii, 22, 58, 77,
129, 130, 219
nitroglycerin, 113–14
nocebo effect, 189–90
noradrenaline (norepinephrine),
xi, 61
Nottingham, University of, 145
nutrition, 228

obesity, 16, 187, 200, 215
Obstetrics & Gynecology, 68
Olivia CD, 24–25, 27, 98, 131
osteoarthritis, 5, 72–73, 165
osteoporosis, 150–51, 230–31
oxidative stress, 23, 29

pacemakers, 43, 66, 218
pain, 147–52
abdominal, 15
acute, 148–49
back, xii, 4–15, 27, 154–55
chronic, xiii, 30, 48, 55, 78, 87,
148, 149
head, 15
joint, 15
mind body approaches to, 7–15,
16, 27, 30, 149–51
neck and shoulder, 15, 16
in phantom limbs, 7, 106
postoperative, 15, 16
standard medical treatments for,
149

pain (*cont.*)
subjectivity of, 148
symptoms of, 147–49
painkillers, 169
pallidotomy, 176
palpitations, 190–97
anxiety and, 118, 119
mind body approaches to, 16,
119, 192–97
standard medical treatments for,
191–92
symptoms of, 190–91
pancreatitis, 154
panic attacks, 55, 118, 179
panic disorder, 118
Parkinson's disease, 16, 176–78
placebo effect and, 48, 85–87,
176–78
standard medical treatment for,
176
symptoms of, 176
Pasteur, Louis, 38–39, 40, 41, 50, 54
penicillin, 17, 43–45
Pennsylvania, University of, 166,
181
performance anxiety, 117–18, 121,
123
perimenopause, 15, 141–42
perspiration, 118, 139
Peru, 34
Peter (patient), 91–93
Peters, Ruanne K., 120
phantom limb pain, 7, 106, 169

phobias, 16, 118, 161, 178–86
mind body approach to, xiii, 16,
180–86
standard medical treatment for,
179–80
symptoms of, 178–79
placebo effect, xi, 8, 52, 56, 76, 77,
78–88, 200, 214
angina pectoris helped by,
79–81, 114–15
blood pressure affected by, 129,
130, 131
for depression, 81–85, 87–88,
125–26
in double-blind controlled
research, 46–48, 86, 214
folk remedies and, 33, 76
for headaches, 160
history of, 45–46, 76
for joint pain, 163
nitric oxide produced by, 77
Parkinson's disease and, 85–87,
176
remembered wellness vs.,
105–6
for sciatica, 157
scientific studies on, 72–73,
78–80, 82, 85–87, 149–52
placebo surgery, 72–73, 80, 85–86,
149–52, 165–66, 167, 230,
231
PLoS ONE, 18, 21
pneumonia, 31–32, 44

positron-emission tomography
(PET), 126
postoperative pain, 15, 16
postoperative swelling, 16, 200
post-traumatic stress disorder
(PTSD), 16, 200
destructive genetic activity and,
24
posture, 137–38
potassium-sparing agents, 129
prayers, 9, 20, 22, 25, 32, 33, 57, 58,
59, 96–97, 111, 115, 222
prefrontal cortex, 187
premature aging, 23, 29, 186–90
mind body approaches to, 16,
187–90
standard medical treatment for,
187
symptoms of, 186
premature ventricular contractions
(PVCs), 115, 190–97
mind body approaches to, 16,
55, 60, 66–68, 192–97, 226
standard medical treatment for,
191–92
symptoms of, 190–91
premenstrual syndrome (PMS),
197–200
mind body approach to, xii, 16,
55, 60, 68–69, 198–200
standard treatment for, 197–98
symptoms of, 197
preventive medicine, 225–27

progesterone, 132–33, 139, 197
progressive muscle relaxation, 57, 97
prosthetic limbs, 43
pruritus, 202, 203
Psychiatry, 57
"psycho-educational interventions,"
142
Psychoneuroendocrinology, 198
Psychotherapy and Psychosomatics,
119

Qigong, 96
quinine, 34

rabies vaccine, 39
Rachel (patient), 31–32
reading, 83–84
recovery, natural course of, 33, 34
reductionism, 74, 208, 211–16, 220,
224
relaxation response, 9–10, 19, 54–
70, 93–99, 108, 110, 111–12,
133, 192, 214, 217, 222, 223
for abdominal pain, 152
for angina pectoris, 116
for anxiety, 118, 120, 121–22,
123
for back pain, 155
for cancer, 203, 204–5, 206
Caroline's use of, 10–12, 13, 27
definition of, 56–59
for depression, 55, 126–27
discovery of, xi, 57–59, 212

relaxation response (*cont.*)
education and, 228–29
eight steps to, 94–95
experience-dependent cortical plasticity and, 187–88
fight-or-flight response vs., xi, 8, 52, 56
for general pain, 152
for general surgery, 174, 175
genetic response and, 10, 24–30, 56, 58–59, 204
for headaches, 55, 159–60, 161–62, 163
for hypertension, 55, 60–64, 128, 129, 130, 190
identification of, 52
for infertility, 55, 60, 69–70, 133
for insomnia, 55, 60, 64–66, 135, 137–38
for irregular heartbeats, 55, 60, 66–68
for joint pain, 164
for menopause, 142, 143
"mini," 115–16, 228
multiple approaches to, 27
for nausea, 146
for neck pain, 168, 169
Olivia CD's similarity to, 27
Peter's use of, 92, 93
for phobias, 182, 185
for PMS, 55, 60, 68–69, 198, 199
for premature aging, 187, 188

PVCs and palpitations and, 195, 196–97
for sciatica, 156
scientific evidence for, 55, 56, 59
for skin cancer, 171, 173
for stress, 56, 57
time for, 9, 19, 110, 227
Relaxation Response, The (Benson and Klipper), 171
relaxation response break, 120
Relaxation Response Milestone, 54, 55–56
Relaxation Response Resiliency Enhancement Programs, 9*n*
relaxation response training diary, 26
religious faith, 32, 33–34, 52, 221–24
remembered wellness, 13–14, 104–5, 127, 138, 143, 153, 155
placebo effect vs., 105–6
repetitive-worship music, 20
respiratory rate, xii
rheumatoid arthritis, 15, 163–64
RICE (rest, ice application, compression, and elevation) treatment, 165
Rigotti, Nancy, 68, 198
Ritalin, 124
rituals, 20
Ron (patient), 156–57

Salisbury, HMS, 35
salt, 68, 128, 197, 226

Samuelson, Marlene, 135, 144

sciatica, 5, 155–56

Science, 57, 61, 213, 217

scurvy, 35–36

Seibel, Machelle M., 69–70

selective serotonin reuptake
  inhibitors (SSRIs), 118, 124,
  125–26, 179, 197

self-esteem, 228

self-hypnosis, 119

Selye, Hans, 52

Semel Institute, UCLA, 104

sepsis, 40

sertraline, 124, 125

sex, sexuality, 65, 124, 228

Shakespeare, William, 71

shock treatments, 125

sick sinus syndrome, 192

side effects, 4, 5, 110, 129, 135, 142,
  179, 215, 218

skin cancer, 170–73

sleep hygiene techniques, 65, 66

sleeping position, 168

sleep medication, 215

sleep onset latency (SOL), 64–65

Slingsby, Brian, 58

smallpox, 36, 37

smoking, 114, 128, 133, 136, 187,
  197, 226

Society for Integrative Oncology,
  205

Southern California, University of,
  193

South Korea, 145

Spain, 37

spinal tumor, 154

Stefano, George, 58

stethoscope, 37

stimulus control, 66, 136–37

streptomycin, 43, 44

stress, 113, 114, 155, 187
  Cannon's investigation of, 52
  chronic pain exacerbated by, 149
  cramps and, 152
  genes and, 15, 23–24, 56, 63–64,
    297
  headaches and, 158
  healing delayed by, 33
  hypertension caused by, 91–92
  infertility caused by, 132–34
  meditation and, 57
  mind body approaches to, 16,
    57, 69, 99, 103, 110, 120–21,
    133, 188, 208, 228
  nausea caused by, 144–45
  oxidative, 23, 29
  and PMS, 198
  PVCs, palpitations and, 195, 196

supportive-expressive group
  intervention, 83, 84

surgery, xii, xiii, 17, 32, 37, 39, 52,
    53, 54, 56, 73, 74, 92, 109,
    110, 225, 229
  antiseptic routine in, 41
  back, 6, 8, 14, 230–31
  for cancer, 43

surgery (*cont.*)
  inert, 72–73, 80, 85–86, 149–52,
    165–66, 167, 230, 231
Sweden, 37
sympathetic nervous system, 57
symptoms, 109–10
synergism, 219–20
systematic desensitization, 145, 182

tachycardia, 169, 191
tai chi, 96
tension headaches, xii, 158, 160
tetanus, 43
thalamotomy, 176
thoughts, obtrusive, 9, 10, 11, 25,
    27
thyroids, 118
time, 110, 227, 230
tinnitus, 16, 200
tranquilizers, 169
Transcendental Meditation, 57, 59,
    62, 96
Transfusion, 181
translational research, 213
trazodone, 124
tuberculosis, 42, 44
typhoid, 40

ulcers, 16, 118

vaccinations, 36, 37, 39
varicoceles, 132
vasodilation, 129, 130

vertebroplasty, 150–51
Vipassana meditation, 59
virtual reality exposure, 180, 182
virus, 44
vis medicatrix naturae, 33
visualization, 9, 10, 19, 99–108,
    110–11, 112, 223, 226
  for abdominal pain, 152–54
  for angina pectoris, 116–17
  for back pain, 154, 155
  Caroline's use of, 12–15
  cognitive behavioral therapy
    and, 106–8
  cognitive restructuring and, 107
  for depression, 127
  desensitization and, 107–8
  for general pain, 152
  for general surgery, 174
  for headaches, 158–63
  for hypertension, 130
  for infertility, 134
  for insomnia, 138
  for joint pain, 163–68
  for menopause, 142, 143
  for nausea, 146
  for neck pain, 168–69
  for Parkinson's disease, 177, 178
  performance paradox of, 101–2
  Peter's use of, 92, 93
  for phobias, 182, 185
  for PMS, 199
  for premature aging, 188, 189
  PVCs, palpitations and, 195–96

Index

for sciatica, 157
for skin cancer, 171, 173
time for, 10, 19, 110, 227
vitamin C, 36
vitamins, 33

weight loss, 114, 124, 128, 133, 154
wellness-based medical model, 106
Wilcher, Marilyn, 228

Wisdom of the Body, The (Cannon), 52
working position, 168
World Health Organization, 38

yoga, 20, 22, 57, 59, 96

Zen, 57
Zusman, Randall, 63